Children, Obesity and Exercise

Prevention, treatment and management of childhood and adolescent obesity

**Edited by Andrew P. Hills,
Neil A. King and
Nuala M. Byrne**

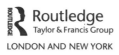 Routledge
Taylor & Francis Group

LONDON AND NEW YORK

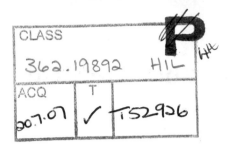
First published 2007
by Routledge
2 Park Square, Milton Park, Abingdon, Oxon OX14 4RN

Simultaneously published in the USA and Canada
by Routledge
270 Madison Ave, New York, NY 10016

Routledge is an imprint of the Taylor & Francis Group, an informa business

© 2007 Selection and editorial material, Andrew P. Hills, Neil A. King and
Nuala M. Byrne, individual contributions, the contributors

Typeset in Goudy by Prepress Projects Ltd, Perth, UK
Printed and bound in Great Britain by TJ International Ltd, Padstow,
Cornwall

British Library Cataloguing in Publication Data
A catalogue record for this book is available from the British Library

Library of Congress Cataloging in Publication Data
Hills, Andrew P.
    Children, obesity & exercise: a practical approach to prevention,
    treatment, and management of childhood and adolescent obesity/
    Andrew P. Hills, Neil A. King & Nuala M. Byrne.
    p.; cm.

    ISBN13: 978–0–415–40883–7 (hbk)
    ISBN10: 0–415–40883–0 (hbk)
    ISBN13: 978–0–415–40884–4 (pbk.)
    ISBN10: 0–415–40884–9 (pbk.)

    1. Obesity in children. 2. Obesity in adolescence. 3. Obesity in children
    – Exercise therapy. 4. Obesity in adolescence – Exercise therapy. I. King,
    Neil A. II. Byrne, Nuala M. III. Title. IV. Title: Children, obesity, and
    exercise.
    [DNLM: 1. Obesity. 2. Adolescent. 3. Child. 4. Exercise. WD 210
    H655e 2007]
    RJ399.C6H55 2007
    618.92´398–dc22
    2007001042

ISBN10: 0–415–40883–0 (hbk)
ISBN10: 0–415–40884–9 (pbk)
ISBN10: 0–203–94597–2 (ebk)
ISBN13: 978–0–415–40883–7 (hbk)
ISBN13: 978–0–415–40884–4 (pbk)
ISBN13: 978–0–203–94597–1 (ebk)

Children, Obesity and Exercise

Throughout the developed world there is an increasing prevalence of childhood obesity. Because of this increase, and awareness of the risks to long-term health that childhood obesity presents, the phenomenon is now described by many as a global epidemic.

Children, Obesity and Exercise provides sport, exercise and medicine students and professionals with an accessible and practical guide to understanding and managing childhood and adolescent obesity. It covers:

- overweight, obesity and body composition;
- physical activity, growth and development;
- psycho-social aspects of childhood obesity;
- physical activity behaviours;
- eating behaviours;
- measuring children's behaviour;
- interventions for prevention and management of childhood obesity.

Children, Obesity and Exercise addresses the need for authoritative advice and innovative approaches to the prevention and management of this chronic problem.

Andrew P. Hills is a Professor in the Institute of Health and Biomedical Information at Queensland University of Technology, Australia.

Neil A. King is in the Institute of Health and Biomedical Information at Queensland University of Technology, Brisbane, Australia.

Nuala M. Byrne is in the Institute of Health and Biomedical Information at Queensland University of Technology, Brisbane, Australia.

International studies in physical education and youth sport
Series Editor: Richard Bailey
Roehampton University, London, UK

Routledge's *International Studies in Physical Education and Youth Sport* series aims to stimulate discussion on the theory and practice of school physical education, youth sport, childhood physical activity and well-being. By drawing on international perspectives, in terms of both the background of the contributors and the selection of the subject matter, the series seeks to make a distinctive contribution to our understanding of issues that continue to attract attention from policy-makers, academics and practitioners.

International Council of Sport Science and Physical Education (ICSSPE)

The International Council of Sport Science and Physical Education (ICSSPE) is an international umbrella organization with a diverse and well-recognized institutional membership worldwide. ICSSPE has formal associate relations with UNESCO, is a recognized organization of the International Olympic Committee (IOC) and cooperates with the World Health Organization (WHO) and other international bodies. ICSSPE promotes and disseminates a wide range of scientific information and facilitates communication between organizations active in the fields of sport, sport science and physical education. ICSSPE's comprehensive website is updated on a regular basis to share knowledge, report events and announce newly published resources. It is just one of the tools ICSSPE uses to build stronger international cooperation and bridge the gap between developed and developing countries.

Since overweight and obesity has become such a critical and multi-faceted issue for all nations it is ICSSPE's aim that all persons, institutes and organizations involved in sport and sport science keep up to date with latest research, strategies and interventions and understand their role in prevention, identification and management of the conditions.

ICSSPE/CIEPSS Executive Office   Tel: +49 30 36 41 88 50
Hanns-Braun-Strasse   Fax: +49 30 805 63 86
Friesenhaus II   Email: icsspe@icsspe.org
14053 Berlin   Internet: www.icsspe.org
Germany

Contents

Figures

Tables

Boxes

Contributors

Louise A. Baur is at the University of Sydney, Sydney, Australia.

Nuala M. Byrne is at Queensland University of Technology, Brisbane, Australia.

Susan Byrne is at the University of Western Australia, Perth, Australia.

Marijke Chin A Paw is at the VU University Medical Centre, The Netherlands.

Tom F. Cuddihy is at Queensland University of Technology, Brisbane, Australia.

Mark Davidson is at Griffith University, Brisbane, Australia.

Ilse De Bourdeaudhuij is at Ghent University, Ghent, Belgium.

Benedicte Deforche is at Ghent University, Ghent, Belgium.

Elizabeth Denney-Wilson is at the University of Sydney, Sydney, Australia.

Helen H.M. Hermsdorff is at the Federal University of Vicosa, Vicosa, Brazil.

Andrew P. Hills is at Queensland University of Technology, Brisbane, Australia.

Masaharu Kagawa is at Queensland University of Technology, Brisbane, Australia.

Neil A. King is at Queensland University of Technology, Brisbane, Australia.

Michelle La Puma is at the University of Western Australia, Perth, Australia.

Linda M. Lyell is at Queensland University of Technology, Brisbane, Australia.

Willem van Mechelen is at the VU University Medical Centre, The Netherlands.

Josefina Bressan is at the Federal University of Vicosa, Vicosa, Brazil.

Robert P. Pangrazi is at Arizona State University, New Mexico, USA.

Amika Singh is at the VU University Medical Centre, The Netherlands.

L. Michaud Tomson is at Griffith University, Brisbane, Australia.

Jos W.R. Twisk is at the VU University Medical Centre, The Netherlands.

Scott C. Wearing is at Queensland University of Technology, Brisbane, Australia.

Jennie Yeung is at Ford Health Group, Brisbane, Australia.

1 Childhood obesity – an introduction

J. Yeung and A.P. Hills

Introduction

The increasing prevalence of childhood overweight and obesity is a global trend (World Health Organization, 1997) and is of concern as overweight or obese children are at a higher risk of experiencing a range of health problems in the immediate, short and long term.

Immediate health problems of overweight and obese children include social isolation and potential psychological dysfunction (Friedman, Story and Perry, 1995; Must, 1996; Must and Strauss, 1999). Young overweight children have been described by their peers as ugly, stupid, dishonest and lazy (Staffieri, 1967) and they may experience teasing and social isolation as a result (Stunkard and Burt, 1967). Such children are also at greater risk of co-morbidities than their lean counterparts. For example, children who are overweight or obese are at greater risk of asthma, and when they have it they have been shown to use more medicine (Belamarich et al., 2000; Luder, Melnik and DiMaio, 1998), wheeze more, experience more unscheduled visits to hospital (Belamarich et al., 2000) and miss more school days as a result of their asthma than lean asthmatic children (Luder, Melnik and DiMaio, 1998).

In the short term, overweight and obese children are more likely to develop certain gastrointestinal, cardiovascular, endocrine and orthopaedic problems than their lean peers that may be exacerbated in the long term. Further, overweight and obese girls are more likely to develop reproductive system abnormalities, such as early onset of puberty and menarche, and polycystic ovary syndrome (Goran, 2001; Must, 1996; Must and Strauss, 1999; Taitz, 1983).

Data from the longitudinal Bogalusa Heart Study suggest that, in the long term, cardiovascular disease risk factor prevalence increases greatly over time in overweight and obese children (Goran, 2001). In short, remaining obese from childhood through adolescence and into adulthood places the individual at a higher risk of associated morbidities (Guo and Chumlea, 1999; Magarey et al., 2003).

Aetiology of obesity

Environmental factors such as diet, physical activity and metabolic status are major contributors to obesity, and in turn are influenced by genetic traits (Weinsier et al., 1998). As a rule, excess body fatness results from a long-term imbalance between energy intake and energy expenditure (NHMRC, 1997).

Diet

The increased consumption of highly refined and often high-fat food products has been identified as a key energy intake factor contributing to overweight and obesity in adults (Popkin, 2001). In Europe and North America, simple sugars and fat account for more than half the energy intake and consumption of refined grains has mostly replaced that of whole grains (Chopra, Galbraith and Darnton-Hill, 2002). Eck et al. (1992) and Gazzaniga and Burns (1993) have reported a significant relationship between childhood obesity and the percentage of dietary intake from fat; however, a study by Wang, Patterson and Hills (2003) found no differences in the average intake of energy and fat between non-overweight and overweight or obese Australian children and adolescents. This finding is consistent with reports from other countries that suggest there has not been a concurrent increase in energy and/or fat intake with increasing obesity prevalence (Nicklas et al., 1993; Rolland-Cachera, Deheeger and Bellisle, 1996).

The apparent lack of consistency in findings for energy and fat intake in youth may be a function of the relative difficulty in accurately measuring individual intake, including reporting biases. More research is required in the area.

Physical activity

In a number of countries, including the United States, there is evidence that physical activity among youth has declined in recent decades and the corresponding increase in obesity prevalence may be the direct result of this decline (Luepker, 1999). An Australian study comparing physical activity in 10- to 11-year-old children from 1985 to 1997 also reported a decrease in physical activity (Dollman et al., 1999).

As for energy intake, the relationship between obesity and physical activity varies across studies. For example some studies (Sunnegardh et al., 1986; Waxman and Stunkard, 1980) have reported an inverse relationship between activity and adiposity levels while others have found no relationship (Saris, 1986; Wilkinson et al., 1977). Again, the measurement challenges in the physical activity area may account for the lack of definitive findings.

Metabolic factors

Weinsier et al. (1998) suggest that a number of metabolic factors have the potential to influence the onset of obesity. These include resting energy expenditure, the thermic effect of food (food- or drink-induced increase in metabolic rate), activity-related energy expenditure and fuel utilization. However, much of the research in this area has been conducted on adults and not the childhood population.

Resting energy expenditure (REE) varies amongst individuals; however, although individual variations in REE may affect total daily energy expenditure, the variations may only have a small impact on the tendency to gain significant weight (Goran *et al.*, 1998; Seidell *et al.*, 1992; Weinsier *et al.*, 1998). Similarly, while the energy expended via the thermic effect of food in obese people may be reduced (Weinsier, Bracco and Schultz, 1993), the potential weight gains are too small to be considered a likely cause of obesity. In contrast, there is widespread acceptance that the most variable component of total energy expenditure, activity energy expenditure (Carpenter *et al.*, 1995; Goran, 1995), is a potentially significant contributor to the predisposition to obesity (Ravussin *et al.*, 1988; Zurlo *et al.*, 1992). The effects, if any, of fuel utilization on obesity are not established (Weinsier *et al.*, 1998).

The impact of the environment in the promotion of childhood obesity

Despite recent advances in genetic research, genetics alone cannot explain the obesity epidemic (Hill and Peters, 1998). Although genetics may predispose some individuals to obesity and related diseases (Carmelli, Cardon and Fabsitz, 1994), this alone is not sufficient to cause the condition (Bouchard, 1995; Greenberg, 1993; Maffeis, 2000) and other determinants must be present for obesity to occur. Eaton, Konner and Shostak (1988a,b) suggest that the human gene pool has not changed substantially over the last 35,000 years but the living environment has been radically transformed, particularly in the past century in industrialized nations.

The 'discordance hypothesis' has been proposed to describe how the human genome, with its various susceptibilities, is more likely to express 'diseases of civilization' in the current environmental circumstances (Eaton, Konner and Shostak, 1988a,b). For example, today, energy-dense foods are readily available and there are commonly minimal requirements for physical activity for subsistence. The hypothesis suggests that obesity results from a mismatch between the modern lifestyle and the lifestyle for which humans, and their genes, evolved. Despite significant advances in reducing mortality related to infectious diseases, detection and treatment of many other conditions and an overall increase in longevity, a shift has occurred to an increase in chronic and degenerative diseases that are strongly associated with the western lifestyle (Popkin, 1998).

Hill and Peters (1998) suggest that the present environment promotes high energy intake and low energy expenditure. Under such circumstances, obesity occurs more frequently because, whereas the body has excellent physiological defence mechanisms that protect against the depletion of body energy stores, it has weak defence mechanisms to prevent the accumulation of excess energy stores when food is abundant. In addition, changes in social eating behaviours, enticing food advertisements and larger food portion sizes may override the normal leptin-induced satiety, and thereby cause excess weight gain.

The term 'obesogenic' has been coined to describe the current environmental circumstances. The obesogenicity of an environment is defined as 'the sum of influences that the surroundings, opportunities, or conditions of life have on promoting obesity in individuals or populations' (Swinburn, Egger and Raza, 1999: 564).

Behavioural determinants of obesity and the effect of the environment

Despite the general consensus that environmental factors are likely to be important in influencing factors such as energy intake, physical activity levels and ultimately body weight, the empirical evidence of a relationship between specific environmental exposures and obesity is poor (Crawford and Ball, 2002). There is a large range of environmental factors that could potentially increase the likelihood of weight gain and thus risk of obesity (Booth et al., 2001; French, Story and Jeffery, 2001), but these environmental influences must be mediated by the population's eating and physical activity behaviours (i.e. through energy intake and energy expenditure) (Crawford and Ball, 2002). These behaviours are critically important since they form the interface between human biology and the environments to which the population is exposed (Crawford and Ball, 2002). In short, the development of obesity may be better understood with knowledge of the population's eating and physical activity behaviours, the determinants of these behaviours, and how they might be influenced (Law, 2001).

From an epidemiological perspective, the behaviours themselves should be focused on, rather than the disease or health condition (Mason and Powell, 1985). Additionally, there should be an examination of their psycho-social and social–ecological antecedents (Raymond, 1989). In relation to obesity, it is important to acknowledge that the environment is but one source of influence, albeit potentially potent (Booth et al., 2001; French, Story and Jeffery, 2001; Kumanyika et al., 2002).

The environment is one of a number of factors that influence obesity development and also affect people's behaviours. Hill and Peters (1998) suggest that the environment's contribution to obesity should be thought of in terms of how it contributes to the frequency of behaviours that increase or decrease the risk of a positive energy balance. For example, parents influence the nature and amount of physical activity in which children engage. Kohl and Hobbs (1998) concluded that parental influence on physical activity among children is most likely an interaction of direct and indirect factors. Parents may have a direct influence by providing an environment that nurtures physical activity in the child, and have indirect influence through modelling of physical activity participation. Young children (four to seven years of age) whose parents were physically active were nearly six times as likely to be physically active as peers of whom neither parent was physically active (Moore et al., 1991). Therefore, parents who provided physical activity-promoting environments, and who were physically active themselves, influenced their children to adopt a significantly higher frequency of physical activity behaviours (and the likelihood of a decreased risk of positive energy balance) compared with children with less physical activity-stimulating environments.

Obesity may thus be viewed as a natural response to the environment. However, within any given environment, an individual has a certain probability of becoming obese but not a certainty. Some individuals resist gaining weight and becoming obese in unsupportive environments by maintaining a pattern of healthy behaviours (Hill and Peters, 1998). Therefore, some individuals are susceptible to the obesogenic environment whilst others are able to resist it.

In summary, obesity is the consequence of an energy imbalance, with energy intake exceeding energy expenditure. Although the expression of certain genes might increase one's vulnerability to obesity, other determinants, a mixture of environmental and behavioural, must be present for obesity to occur.

Necessary modifications to the environment to afford a shift in activity levels

From research evidence to date, Campbell *et al.* (2002) believe that childhood obesity prevention strategies should encourage a reduction in sedentary behaviours with concurrent increases in physical activity. Advances in technology and transportation have reduced the need for physical activity in daily life (Hill and Peters, 1998), and the appeal of television, electronic games and computers has increased the time spent in sedentary pursuits among both children and adults. If a low level of physical activity energy expenditure is not matched with a correspondingly lower daily energy requirement, weight gain is the likely outcome.

An important challenge is to provide all children with an environment conducive to regular physical activity. This is particularly difficult given the diversity of urban and rural settings and mix of socioeconomic determinants. For example, a study of a multiethnic sample of youth indicated that racial/ethnic disparities in exercise levels were mediated by disparities in access to exercise facilities and programmes (Garcia *et al.*, 1995). A parallel challenge is to encourage all children to be physically active irrespective of size, shape and physical ability (Hills and Cambourne, 2002).

Investigations using self-report and/or more objective measures of physical activity have identified the following correlates of physical activity behaviour: physical activity self-efficacy (Trost *et al.*, 1996, 1997, 1999); enjoyment (Borra *et al.*, 1995; Stucky-Ropp and DiLorenzo, 1993); parental influences (Moore *et al.*, 1991; Sallis *et al.*, 1992); attitudes or beliefs about physical activity outcomes (Craig, Goldberg and Dietz, 1996; Theodorakis *et al.*, 1991; Trost *et al.*, 1999); access to equipment and programmes (Pate *et al.*, 1997; Trost *et al.*, 1997); social norms regarding physical activity (Trost *et al.*, 1999); involvement in community-based physical activity organizations (Trost *et al.*, 1999); and time spent outdoors (Trost *et al.*, 1999).

The most salient predictor of exercise behaviour was child enjoyment of physical activity (Stucky-Ropp and DiLorenzo, 1993). Poor physical activity experiences may be a significant contributor to reduced levels of physical activity and, consequently, problems in the maintenance of energy balance (Hills and Cambourne, 2002). Therefore, physical activity experiences for children must be positive and conducted in a manner that fosters fun and enjoyment. Success in the activity setting is a major determinant of continued participation in activity as success affects self-efficacy. As a consequence, to maximize habitual physical activity in youngsters, they need to experience a measure of success and a sense of belonging. The goal for each individual should be to participate in physical activity at every opportunity.

Role of different settings

Schools are a natural setting to influence the physical activity behaviours of young people (Resnicow and Robinson, 1997). Traditionally, physical activity opportunities were provided for many children in the context of physical education programmes; however, quality programmes are now the exception rather than the rule. Increases in current sports participation and/or physical education time at school would require policy changes at both the school and education department levels. Similarly, increases in active modes of transport to and from school (walking, cycling and public transport) would be contingent upon policy changes at school and local government levels, in addition to support from parents and members of the wider community (Swinburn and Egger, 2002).

Strategies are needed to allow children the freedom to walk and cycle to and from school. Schemes that provide safe routes to school or 'walking buses'/walk-to-school programmes therefore appear well founded at this point. Similarly, well-designed playgrounds, cycle paths and storage space for bicycles are important.

The home environment is another critical setting in which the 'activity ethos' of the family underpins participation and beliefs (Swinburn and Egger, 2002). Parents play important health-related roles for their children and should ideally be models of appropriate behaviour and major sources of reinforcement in the lives of children (Perry *et al.*, 1988). Parents may be considered as gatekeepers, providing opportunities and/or barriers to physical activity of their children.

An associated factor in the physical activity participation of many families is the provision of recreational facilities, which is the core business of local governments (Swinburn and Egger, 2002). Recreational spaces may be enhanced by local government in a variety of ways such as extending walking and cycle paths; the addition of facilities including skateboard ramps; increasing lighting and attractiveness of spaces; and also contributing to a reduction in crime rates in the area. In established residential areas it is difficult to increase the amount of open recreational space. An allied problem may be the protection of green spaces that may be compromised through commercial pressures (Swinburn and Egger, 2002).

References

Belamarich, P.F., Luder, E., Kattan, M., Mitchell, H., Islam, S., Lynn, H. and Crain, E.F. (2000) 'Do obese inner-city children with asthma have more symptoms than nonobese children with asthma?', *Pediatrics*, 106: 1436–42.

Booth, S.L., Sallis, J.F., Ritenbaugh C., Hill, J.O., Birch L.L., Frank, L.D., Glanz, K., Himmelgreen, D.A., Mudd, M., Popkin, B.M., Rickard, K.A., St. Jeor, S. and Hays, N.P. (2001) 'Environmental and societal factors affect food choice and physical activity: rationale, influences and leverage points', *Nutrition Review*, 59: S21–39.

Borra, S.T., Schwartz, N.E., Spain, C.G. and Natchipolsky, M.M. (1995) 'Food, physical activity, and fun: inspiring America's kids to more healthy lifestyles', *Journal of the American Dietetic Association*, 95: 816–18.

Bouchard, C. (1995) 'Genetics of obesity: an update on molecular markers', *International Journal of Obesity*, 19(Suppl 3): S10–13.

Campbell, K., Waters, E., O'Meara, S., Kelly, S. and Summerbell, C. (2002) 'Interventions for preventing obesity in children', *Cochrane Database of Systematic Reviews*, CD001871.

Carmelli, D., Cardon, L.R. and Fabsitz, R. (1994) 'Clustering of hypertension, diabetes and obesity in adult male twins: same genes or same environments?', *American Journal of Human Genetics*, 55: 566–73.

Carpenter, W.H., Poehlman, E.T., O'Connell, M. and Goran, M.I. (1995) 'Influence of body composition and resting metabolic rate on variation in total energy expenditure: a meta analysis', *American Journal of Clinical Nutrition*, 61: 4–10.

Chopra, M., Galbraith, S. and Darnton-Hill, I. (2002) 'A global response to a global problem: the epidemic of overnutrition', *Bulletin: World Health Organization*, 80: 952–58.

Craig, S., Goldberg, J. and Dietz, W.H. (1996) 'Psychosocial correlates of physical activity among fifth and eighth graders', *Preventative Medicine*, 25: 506–18.

Crawford, D. and Ball, K. (2002) 'Behavioural determinants of the obesity epidemic', *Asia Pacific Journal of Clinical Nutrition*, 11(Suppl 8): S718–21.

Dollman, J., Olds, T., Norton, K. and Stuart, D. (1999) 'The evolution of fitness and fatness in 10–11-year-old Australian schoolchildren: changes in distributional characteristics between 1985 and 1997', *Pediatric Exercise Science*, 11: 108–21.

Eaton, S.B., Konner, M. and Shostak, M. (1988a) 'Stone agers in the fast lane: chronic degenerative diseases in evolutionary perspective', *American Journal of Medicine*, 84: 739–49.

Eaton, S.B., Konner, M. and Shostak, M. (1988b) *The Paleolithic Prescription*, New York: Harper & Row.

Eck, L.H., Klesges, R.C., Hanson, C.L. and Slawson, D. (1992) 'Children at familial risk for obesity: an examination of dietary intake, physical activity and weight status', *International Journal of Obesity*, 16: 71–8.

French, S.A., Story, M. and Jeffery, R.W. (2001) 'Environmental influences on eating and physical activity', *Annual Review of Public Health*, 22: 309–35.

Friedman, S.A., Story, M. and Perry, C.L. (1995) 'Self-esteem and obesity in children and adolescents: a literature review', *Obesity Research*, 3: 479–90.

Garcia, A.W., Broda, M.A., Frenn, M., Coviak, C., Pender, N.J. and Ronis, D.L. (1995) 'Gender and developmental differences in beliefs among youth and prediction of their exercise behavior', *Journal of School Health*, 65: 213–20.

Gazzaniga, J.M. and Burns, T.L. (1993) 'Relationship between diet composition and body fatness, with adjustment for resting energy expenditure and physical activity, in pre-adolescent children', *American Journal of Clinical Nutrition*, 58: 21–8.

Goran, M.I. (1995) 'Variation in total energy expenditure in humans', *Obesity Research*, 3: 59–66.

Goran, M.I. (2001) 'Metabolic precursors and effects of obesity in children: a decade of progress, 1990–1999', *American Journal of Clinical Nutrition*, 73: 158–71.

Goran, M.I., Shewchuk, R., Gower, B.A., Nagy, T.R., Carpenter, W.H. and Johnson, R.K. (1998) 'Longitudinal changes in fatness in white children: no effect of childhood energy expenditure', *American Journal of Clinical Nutrition*, 67: 309–16.

Greenberg, D.A. (1993) 'Linking analysis of "necessary" disease loci versus "susceptibility" loci', *American Journal of Human Genetics*, 52: 135–43.

Guo, S.S. and Chumlea, W.C. (1999) 'Tracking of body mass index in children in relation to overweight in adulthood', *American Journal of Clinical Nutrition*, 70: 145–8.

Hill, J.O. and Peters, J.C. (1998) 'Environmental contributions to the obesity epidemic', *Science*, 280: 1371–4.

Hills, A.P. and Cambourne, B. (2002) 'Walking to school – a sustainable environmental strategy to prevent childhood obesity', *Australian Epidemiologist*, 9: 15–18.

Kohl, H.W. III and Hobbs, K.E. (1998) 'Development of physical activity behaviors among children and adolescents', *Pediatrics*, 101: 549–54.

Kumanyika, S., Jeffery, R.W., Morabia, A., Rittenbaugh, C. and Antipastis, V. (2002) 'Obesity prevention: the case for action', *International Journal of Obesity*, 26: 425–6.

Law, C. (2001) 'Adult obesity and growth in childhood: children who grow rapidly during childhood are more likely to be obese as adults', *British Medical Journal*, 323: 1320–1.

Luder, E, Melnik, T.A. and DiMaio, M. (1998) 'Association of being overweight with greater asthma symptoms in inner city black and Hispanic children', *Journal of Pediatrics*, 132: 699–703.

Luepker, R.V. (1999) 'How physically active are American children and what can we do about it?', *International Journal of Obesity*, 23(Suppl 2): S12–17.

Maffeis, C. (2000) 'Aetiology of overweight and obesity in children and adolescents', *European Journal of Pediatrics*, 159(Suppl 1): S35–44.

Magarey, A.L., Daniels, L.A., Boulton, T.J.C. and Cockington, R.A. (2003) 'Predicting obesity in early adulthood from childhood and parental obesity', *International Journal of Obesity*, 27: 505–13.

Mason, J.P. and Powell, K.E. (1985) 'Physical activity, behavioral epidemiology, and public health', *Public Health Reports*, 100: 113–15.

Moore, L.L., Lombardi, D.A., White, M.J., Campbell, J.L., Oiveria, S.A. and Ellison, R.C. (1991) 'Influence of parents' physical activity levels on activity levels of young children', *Journal of Pediatrics*, 118: 215–19.

Must, A. (1996) 'Morbidity and mortality associated with elevated body weight in children and adolescents', *American Journal of Clinical Nutrition*, 63: S445–7.

Must, A. and Strauss, R.S. (1999) 'Risks and consequences of childhood and adolescent obesity', *International Journal of Obesity*, 23(Suppl 2): S2–11.

NHMRC (National Health and Medical Research Council) (1997) *Acting on Australia's Weight: A Strategic Plan for the Prevention of Overweight and Obesity*, Canberra: Australian Government Publishing Service.

Nicklas, T.A., Webber, L.S., Srinivasan, S.R. and Berenson, G.S. (1993) 'Secular trends in dietary intakes and cardiovascular risk factors of 10-y-old children: the Bogalusa Heart Study', *American Journal of Clinical Nutrition*, 57: 930–7.

Pate, R.R., Trost, S.G., Felton, G.M., Ward, D.S., Dowda, M. and Saunders, R. (1997) 'Correlates of physical activity behavior in rural youth', *Research Quarterly for Exercise and Sport*, 68: 241–8.

Perry, C.L., Luepker, R.V., Murray, D.M., Kurth, C., Mullis, R., Crockett, S. and Jacobs, D.R., Jr (1988) 'Parent involvement with children's health promotion: the Minnesota Home Team', *American Journal of Public Health*, 78: 1156–60.

Popkin, B.M. (1998) 'The nutrition transition and its health implications in lower-income countries', *Public Health Nutrition*, 1: 5–21.

Popkin, B.M. (2001) 'Nutrition in transition: the changing global nutrition challenge', *Asia Pacific Journal of Clinical Nutrition*, 101: S13–18.

Ravussin, E., Lillioja, S. Knowler, W.C., Christin, L., Freymond, D., Abbott, W.G., Boyce, V., Howard, B.V. and Bogardus, C. (1988) 'Reduced rate of energy expenditure as a risk factor for body-weight gain', *New England Journal of Medicine*, 318: 467–72.

Raymond, J.S. (1989) 'Behavioral epidemiology: the science of health promotion', *Health Promotion*, 4: 281–6.

Resnicow, K. and Robinson, T.N. (1997) 'School-based cardiovascular disease prevention studies: review and synthesis', *Annals of Epidemiology*, 7: S14–31.

Rolland-Cachera, M.F., Deheeger, M. and Bellisle, F. (1996) 'Nutritional changes between 1978 and 1995 in 10 year-old French children', *International Journal of Obesity*, 20: 53.

Sallis, J.F., Alcaraz, J.E., McKenzie, T.L., Hovell, M.F., Kolody, B. and Nader, P.R. (1992) 'Parental behavior in relation to physical activity and fitness in 9-year-old children', *American Journal of Diseases of Children*, 146: 1383–8.

Saris, W.H.M. (1986) 'Habitual physical activity in children: methodology and findings in health and disease', *Medicine and Science in Sports Exercise*, 18: 253–63.

Seidell, J.C., Muller, D.C., Sorkin, J.D. and Andres, R. (1992) 'Fasting respiratory exchange ratio and resting metabolic rate as predictors of weight gain: the Baltimore Longitudinal Study on Aging', *International Journal of Obesity*, 16: 667–74.

Staffieri, J.R. (1967) 'A study of social stereotype and of body image in children', *Journal of Personality and Social Psychology*, 7: 101–4.

Stucky-Ropp, R. and DiLorenzo, T. (1993) 'Determinants of exercise in children', *Preventative Medicine*, 22: 880–9.

Stunkard, A. and Burt, V. (1967). 'Obesity and the body image: II. Age at onset of disturbances in the body image', *American Journal of Psychiatry*, 123: 1443–7.

Sunnegardh, J., Bratteby, L.E, Hagman, U., Samuelson, G. and Sjolin, S. (1986) 'Physical activity in relation to energy intake and body fat in 8 and 13-year-old children in Sweden', *Acta Paediatrica*, 75: 955–63.

Swinburn, B. and Egger, G. (2002) 'Preventive strategies against weight gain and obesity', *Obesity Reviews*, 3: 289–301.

Swinburn, B., Egger, G. and Raza, F. (1999) 'Dissecting obesogenic environments: the development and application of a framework for identifying and prioritizing environmental interventions for obesity', *Preventative Medicine*, 29: 563–70.

Taitz, L.S. (1983) *The Obese Child*, Boston, MA: Blackwell Scientific Publications.

Theodorakis, Y., Doganis, G., Bagiatis, K. and Gouthas, M. (1991) 'Preliminary study of the ability of reasoned action model in predicting exercise behavior of young children', *Perceptual and Motor Skills*, 72: 51–8.

Trost, S.G., Pate, R.R., Dowda, M., Saunders, R., Ward, D.S. and Felton, G. (1996) 'Gender differences in physical activity and determinants of physical activity in rural fifth grade children', *Journal of School Health*, 66: 145–50.

Trost, S.G., Pate, R.R., Saunders, R., Ward, D.S., Dowda, M. and Felton, G. (1997) 'A prospective study of the determinants of physical activity behaviour in rural fifth-grade children', *Preventative Medicine*, 27: 257–63.

Trost, S.G., Pate, R.R., Ward, D.S., Saunders, R. and Riner, W. (1999) 'Correlates of objectively measured physical activity in preadolescent youth', *American Journal of Preventative Medicine*, 17: 120–6.

Wang, Z., Patterson, C.M. and Hills, A.P. (2003) 'The relationship between BMI and intake of energy and fat in Australian youth: a secondary analysis of the National Nutrition Survey 1995', *Nutrition & Dietetics*, 60: 23–9.

Waxman, M. and Stunkard, A.J. (1980) 'Caloric intake and expenditure of obese boys', *Journal of Pediatrics*, 96: 187–93.

Weinsier, R.L., Bracco, D. and Shultz, Y. (1993) 'Predicted effects of small decreases in energy expenditure on weight gain in adult women', *International Journal of Obesity*, 17: 693–700.

Weinsier, R.L., Hunter, G.R., Heini, A.F., Goran, A.I. and Sell, S.M. (1998) 'The aetiology of obesity: relative contribution of metabolic factors, diet, and physical activity', *American Journal of Medicine*, 105: 145–50.

Wilkinson, P.W., Parkin, J.M., Pearlson, G., Strong, M. and Sykes, P. (1977) 'Energy intake and physical activity in obese children', *British Medical Journal*, 1: 756.

World Health Organization (1997) *Obesity, Preventing and Managing the Global Epidemic: Report of the WHO Consultation of Obesity*, Geneva: World Health Organization.

Zurlo, F., Ferraro, R.T., Fontvielle, A.M., Rising, R., Bogardus, C. and Ravussin, E. (1992) 'Spontaneous physical activity and obesity: cross-sectional and longitudinal studies in Pima Indians', *American Journal of Physiology*, 263: 296–300.

2 Tracking of overweight and obesity from childhood into adulthood

Health consequences and implications for further research

M.J.M. Chin A Paw, A.S. Singh,
J.W.R. Twisk and W. van Mechelen

Introduction

Available prevalence data show that childhood overweight and obesity are increasing dramatically, both in the developed world and in many developing countries (Livingstone, 2001; Martorell *et al.*, 2000; Reilly, 2005). The overweight epidemic in children is alarming because of the clinical and public health implications at young and older ages. Although overweight and obesity in adulthood are clearly linked to an increased risk for morbidity and mortality (Peeters *et al.*, 2003), the long-term health consequences and risks of childhood obesity are less clear.

Identification and targeting preventive efforts at children who are at greatest risk of future obesity is a sensible strategy, but this assumes that obese children have a strong tendency to become obese adults (tracking of obesity). The aim of this chapter is to summarize available data on tracking of overweight and obesity from childhood into adulthood. Furthermore, the long-term health consequences of childhood obesity are reviewed.

Defining overweight and obesity

The World Health Organization guidelines define adults with a body mass index (BMI) of 25 kg/m^2 or more as overweight and those with a BMI of 30 kg/m^2 or more as obese (WHO, 1998). These cut-off points are related to health risks among adults. BMI is a practical and easily computed indicator of relative weight and is highly correlated with more direct measures of fatness (Casey *et al.*, 1992). However, a limitation of using BMI as a measure of body fatness is that BMI reflects both lean and fat mass. Since the BMI is lower in children and adolescents than in adults, the abovementioned definitions are not suitable for the younger age groups. BMI changes during childhood and differs between boys and girls, so age- and sex-specific reference data are necessary.

Cole *et al.* (2000) presented age- and sex-specific cut-off points from 2 to 18 years to define childhood obesity based on pooled international data for BMI and linked to the widely used adult obesity cut-off points of 25 and 30 kg/m². Unfortunately, in earlier studies a wide variety of definitions of child obesity have been used. Percentiles such as the eighty-fifth have commonly been used but the value of this cut-off depends upon the sample on which it was based. Increasing levels of obesity in populations means that the eighty-fifth percentile has also increased, leading to different cut-off points for different time periods as well as for different populations.

Tracking of overweight and obesity from childhood into adulthood

In the epidemiological literature, tracking is used to describe the relative stability of the longitudinal development of a certain outcome variable. The following concepts are usually involved: (1) the relationship (correlation) between early measurements and measurements later in life, or the maintenance of a relative position within a distribution of values in the observed population over time, and (2) the predictability of future values by early measurements (Twisk, Kemper and Mellenbergh, 1994; Ware and Wu, 1981). In epidemiology, tracking mainly refers to the assessment of risk factors for chronic diseases (Twisk, Mechelen and Kemper, 2000). With regard to the possibility of early detection and treatment of overweight and obesity, the assessment of the relationship between childhood weight status and both adult weight status as well as risk factors for chronic disease at any given age are very important. A strong relationship means that it is possible to identify groups with a high probability of overweight in adulthood for which intervention programmes may be implemented.

Table 2.1 presents a summary of studies on tracking of childhood weight for height into adulthood. Eighteen studies are presented, with seven studies following the subjects from birth to young adulthood, and three obtaining data within the first two years of life. Eleven of these studies followed their subjects up to age 30 years or older. Most studies reported only weak to moderate associations between BMI in childhood and BMI in adulthood. Correlations between BMI between the ages of 13–15 years and 20–50 years vary from 0.39 to 0.85; correlations between the ages 17–18 years and 21–40 vary from 0.56 to 0.86. Odds ratios for obesity in adulthood vary from 3.0 to 8.8 at age 6–9 years and from 4.3 to 17.5 at age 15–17 years. All studies found that tracking was stronger for shorter age intervals. Thus, the probability of overweight dependent on childhood values increases with childhood age. Some studies found more consistency in BMI from childhood to adulthood for females than for males (Braddon *et al.*, 1986; Guo *et al.*, 1994; Lake, Power and Cole, 1997) but contrary findings have also been reported (Williams, 2001).

Parental obesity significantly alters the risk of obesity in adulthood for both obese and non-obese children. Subjects with two obese parents show the strongest pattern of tracking of obesity from childhood to adulthood (Lake, Power and Cole, 1997; Whitaker *et al.*, 1997).

Table 2.1 Summary of studies on tracking of overweight from childhood to adulthood

Author	N	Age at inclusion	Follow-up	Outcome measure	Tracking coefficient
Braddon et al. (1986)	3,280	Birth	36 y	BMI	Correlations (m/f)[a]: from 7 y to 20 y–26 y–36 y: 0.41–0.33–0.28/0.47–0.40–0.40 from 11 y to 20 y–26 y–36 y: 0.54–0.46–0.45/0.58–0.51–0.51 from 14 y to 20 y–26 y–36 y: 0.57–0.52–0.46/0.71–0.64–0.60
Casey et al. (1992)	134	Birth	50 y	BMI	Correlations (m/f)[a]: childhood to 18–50 y: 0.36–0.44/0.03–0.53 early adolescence to 18–50 y: 0.47–0.62/0.25–0.82 age of peak height velocity to 18–50 y: 0.55–0.65/0.35–0.84 late adolescence to 18–50 y: 0.55–0.79/0.26–0.85
Guo et al. (1994)	555	1 y	35 y	BMI	ORs[b] (95% CI)[c] for adults at 35 y (childhood BMI 75th percentile vs. 50th percentile) (m/f)[a]: 3y: 1.48 (0.99, 2.21)/1.54 (1.01, 2.35) 8 y: 2.43 (1.50, 3.92)/3.06 (1.72, 5.46) 13 y: 3.26 (2.03, 5.23)/2.44 (1.54, 3.89) 18 y: 9.49 (4.00, 22.51)/5.80 (2.90, 11.63)
Lake et al. (1997)	12,747	Birth	33 y	EMI	Correlations (m/f)[a]: from 7 y to 33 y (both parents non-obese): 0.25/0.32 from 7 y to 33 y (both parents obese): 0.46/0.54
Whitaker et al. (1997)	854	1–2 y	29 y	EMI	ORs[b] for obesity in adulthood: yes vs. not obese/2 vs. 0 parents obese: from 1–2 y to 29 y: 1.3/13.6 from 3–5 y to 29 y: 4.7/15.3 from 6–9 y to 29 y: 8.8/5.0 from 10–14 y to 29 y: 22.3/2.0 from 15–17y to 29 y: 17.5/5.6

Table 2.1 Continued

Author	N	Age at inclusion	Follow-up	Outcome measure	Tracking coefficient
van Lenthe et al. (1996)	500	13 y	29 y	Single trunk and extremity skinfolds	*Correlations (m/f)[a]:* 0.35–0.54/0.31–0.48 *Longitudinal tracking coefficients (association between initial measurement with all other periods of measurement) (m/f)[a]:* 0.56–0.67/0.57–0.70
Laitinen et al. (2001)	12,068	1 y	31y	BMI	*Association between BMI at 14 y and 31 y, regression coefficient (95% CI)[c] (m/f)[a]* [adjusted for maternal BMI, age, social class, and birth weight]: 0.71 (0.67, 0.76)/1.02 (0.96, 1.07)
Hulens et al. (2001)	161 boys	13 y	40 y	BMI	*Correlations:* from 13 y to 18/40 y: 0.77/0.49 from 17 y to 40 y: 0.56
Wright et al. (2001)	412	Birth	50 y	BMI % body fat	*Correlations:* BMI: from 9 y/13 y to 50: 0.24/0.39 % body fat: from 9 y/13 y to 50 y: 0.10/0.22
Williams (2001)	339–500	3 y	21 y	BMI	*Correlations (m/f)[a]:* from 11 y to 21 y: 0.68/0.60 from 13 y to 21 y: 0.71/0.62 from 15 y to 21 y: 0.76/0.69 from 18 y to 21 y: 0.86/0.64
Eriksson et al. (2001) and	3,659	Birth	adult	BMI (adult height and weight self-reported)	OR[b] (95% CI)[c] (m/f)[a] [age-adjusted for adult obesity according to BMI at age 7 y for children with a BMI > 16]: 3.0 (2.2, 4.2)/3.0 (2.3, 3.9)
Eriksson et al. (2003)	4,515	Birth	56–66 y		OR[b] for adult obesity [age-adjusted]: 6.4 (highest ponderal index at birth and BMI at 11 y compared to those with lowest ponderal index at birth and BMI at 11 y)

Study	N			Measure	Results
Trudeau et al. (2001)	191	10–12 y	34 y	BMI, sum of four skinfolds	*Correlation coefficients (m/f)[a]:* BMI: 0.43–0.49/0.64–0.70 sum of four skinfolds: 0.23–0.56/0.45–0.61
Kvaavik, Tell and Klepp (2003)	485	15 y	32 y	BMI (adult height and weight self-reported)	*Correlation: (both genders combined):* 0.54
Magarey et al. (2003)	155	Birth	20 y	BMI	*Correlations:* from 2 y/6 y/11 y/15 y to 20 y: 0.44/0.61/0.72/0.80 RR[d] of overweight at age 20 y (95% CI)[c]: 8 y: 3.47 (2.41, 5.01) 15 y: 4.28 (3.01, 6.08)
Oren et al. (2003)	750	14 y	28 y	BMI	*Correlations (m/f)[a]:* 0.62/0.65
Raitakari et al. (2003)	2,229	3–18 y	32 y	BMI	*Regression coefficients (SE)[e] (m/f)[a]:* 0.013 (0.005)/–0.014 (0.004)
Boreham et al. (2004)	476	15 y	22 y	BMI, sum of four skinfolds	*Kappa's (m/f)[a]:* BMI: 0.42/0.45 sum of four skinfolds: 0.22/0.36
Juonala et al. (2006)	2,260	3–18 y	24–39 y	BMI	*Correlations (both genders combined):* 0.30–0.65
Deshmukh-Taskar et al. (2006)	841	10 y	28 y	BMI	*Correlation:* 0.66 *Kappa's (BMI quartile status) (m/f)[a]:* Euro-American: 0.27/0.23 Afro-American: 0.27/0.35

Notes

a, male/female; b, odds ratio; c, 95% confidence interval; d, relative risk; e, standard error

Table 2.2 Summary of studies on health consequences of childhood overweight

Author	N	Age at inclusion/ measurements during childhood and adolescence/ time interval follow-up	Outcome measures	Results
Mossberg (1989)	504 overweight children included between 1921 and 1947	0–16 y/10 y intervals/40 y	Difference percentage morbidity	*Difference (study population/reference population)*: cardiovascular disease: 29.1%/14.7% diabetes: 7.4%/2.3% digestive disease: 15.3%/4.0% hypertension: 13.6%/8.1% locomotor disease: 19.1%/12.9%
Nieto, Szklo and Comstock (1992)	13,146 subjects included between 1933 and 1945	5–18 y/–/40–52 y	Adult mortality risk for subjects in the top quintile of relative weight	ORs[a] *(m/f/both genders combined)* *(95% CI)*[c]: prepubertal: 1.5 (0.9, 2.7)/1.5 (0.8, 3.1)/1.5 (1.0, 2.4) postpubertal: 1.2 (0.6, 2.2)/2.0 (1.1, 3.6)/1.6 (1.0, 2.4)
Must *et al.* (1992)	508 subjects included between 1922 and 1935	13–18 y/annual measurements until graduation/55 y	mortality risk and morbidity risk	RR[d] [adjusted for adult BMI]: *mortality (95% CI) (both genders combined/m/f)*[b]: all causes: 1.8 (1.2, 2.7)/1.0 (0.6, 1.6) coronary heart disease: 2.3 (1.4, 4.1)/0.8 (0.3, 2.1) cerebrovascular disease: 13.2 (1.6, 108.0)/0.4 (0.1, 1.8) colorectal cancer: 9.1 (1.1, 77.5)/1.0 (0.1, 7.0) breast cancer: –/0.9 (0.2, 3.8) *morbidity (95% CI)*[c] *(m/f)*[b]: coronary heart disease: 1.8 (0.9, 3.9)/2.5 (0.9, 7.1)/1.4 (0.5, 4.0) angina pectoris: 1.5 (0.6, 4.1)/1.3 (0.4, 3.9)/3.7 (0.4, 37.4) diabetes mellitus: 1.0 (0.5, 2.3)/0.9 (0.3, 2.6)/1.2 (0.3, 4.3) atherosclerosis: 7.3 (0.3, 68.3)/3.4 (0.3, 39.2)/infinite stroke: 1.1 (0.3, 4.5)/0.8 (0.1, 5.3)/2.0 (0.1, 28.9) colorectal cancer: 5.6 (0.6, 57.5) (men accounted for all cases) arthritis: 1.2 (0.7, 2.0)/0.7 (0.3, 1.7)/1.6 (0.8, 3.2) gout 2.7 (0.9, 8.4)/2.2 (0.7, 6.9)/infinite

Reference	Subjects	Age/follow-up	Outcome	Results
Lake, Power and Cole (1997)	5,799 female subjects, born in 1958	Birth/7 y, 11 y, 16y/23 y and 33 y	Risk to reproductive health in women at age 33 years according to childhood weight status	ORs[a]: menstrual problems: 1.78 hypertension in pregnancy: 1.46 (overweight) and 2.14 (obese)
Gunnell et al. (1998)	1,165 male and 1,234 female subjects, included between 1937 and 1939	2–14 y/–/57 y	Risk for all death causes, all cardiovascular risks, ischaemic heart disease for children above the 75th percentile	Hazard ratios (95% CI)[c] (m/f/both gender combined)[b]: all-cause mortality: 1.6 (1.0, 2.5)/1.5 (0.8, 2.8)/1.6 (1.1, 2.3) all cardiovascular deaths: 1.9 (1.0, 3.6)/0.9 (0.3, 3.2)/1.6 (0.9, 2.7) ischaemic heart disease: 2.7 (1.2, 6.0)/0.5 (0.1, 4.5)/2.0 (1.0, 3.9) stroke: –/–/1.3 (0.3, 5.0) [using z scores for BMI]
Vanhala et al. (1998)	1,008 subjects born in the years 1947, 1952 and 1957	Birth/age 7 y/36–46 y	Risk for metabolic syndrome for subjects who had been obese as children	OR[a] (95% CI)[c]: 2.9 (1.1, 7.6)
Freedman et al. (2001)	2,617 subjects included between 1973 and 1974	5–17 y/after 9, 12, 15 and 18 years/22 y	Association between BMI and total cholesterol, triglycerides, LDL cholesterol, HDL cholesterol, insulin, systolic blood pressure, diastolic blood pressure	Regression coefficients for childhood BMI [adjusted for adult BMI]: total cholesterol: –0.08 triglycerides: –0.09 LDL cholesterol: –0.09 HDL cholesterol: 0.07 insulin: –0.15 systolic blood pressure: –0.07 diastolic blood pressure: –0.05

Table 2.2 Continued

Author	N	Age at inclusion/ measurements during childhood and adolescence/ time interval follow-up	Outcome measures	Results
Wright et al (2001)	412 subjects, born in 1947	Birth/age 9 y and 13 y/37 y	Association between BMI and total cholesterol, triglyceride concentration	Regression coefficients (females age 9 y/females age 13 y/males age 9 y/males age 13 y) [adjusted for percentage body fat at age 50 years]: carotid thickness: 0.01/0.11/−0.04/−0.07 systolic blood pressure: −0.08/−0.01/0.01/0.04 diastolic blood pressure: −0.08/−0.04/0.01/−0.06 fibrinogen: −0.08/−0.11/−0.004/0.13 total cholesterol: −0.17/−0.16/−0.02/−0.02 HDL cholesterol: −0.08/−0.11/−0.01/−0.09 LDL cholesterol: −0.14/−0.13/−0.03/−0.06 triglyceride: −0.21/−0.12/−0.06/−0.001 2 hour glucose: −0.14/−0.16/−0.12/0.01 serum insulin: −0.12/−0.08/−0.03/−0.08
Oren et al. (2003)	750 subjects, born between 1970 and 1973	Age 12–16 y/–/27–30 y	Association between BMI and carotid intima-media thickness	Regression coefficients (95%CI)[c] [adjusted for adolescent age, gender, lumen diameter, adolescent blood pressure, and puberty stage]: 2.3 (1.3, 3.3) [additionally adjusted for adult blood pressure, adult LDL-cholesterol, and adult BMI]: 0.9 (−0.3, 2.2)

Reference	Sample	Age at measurement/follow-up	Association studied	Regression coefficients (SE)[e] (m/f)[b]:
Raitakari et al. (2003)	2,229 born between 1962 and 1977	3–18 y/after 3 and 6 years/24–39 y	Association between BMI and carotid artery intima-media thickness and total cholesterol, LDL cholesterol, HDL cholesterol, LDL/HDL ratio, triglycerides, systolic blood pressure, diastolic blood pressure	total cholesterol: 0.017 (0.005)/0.004 (0.004) LDL cholesterol: 0.017 (0.005)/0.005 (0.005) HDL cholesterol: −0.001 (0.005)/−0.004 (0.004) LDL/HDL ratio: 0.026 (0.005)/0.007 (0.004) triglycerides: 0.012 (0.005)/0.007 (0.004) systolic blood pressure: 0.020 (0.005)/0.012 (0.004) diastolic blood pressure: 0.011 (0.005)/0.002 (0.004)

Notes

a, odds ratio; b, male/female; c, 95% confidence interval; d, relative risk; e, standard error

Childhood obesity and long-term health consequences

The dramatic increase in the prevalence of childhood obesity within the last decade has changed the view on childhood obesity and the condition is now seen as one of the top 10 global health problems (WHO, 1998). The consequences of obesity in adulthood are well documented and include increased incidence of hypertension, type 2 diabetes, dyslipidaemia and increased risk for certain cancers (Must and Strauss, 1999). See Chapter 3 for further details of the clinical correlates of obesity. The short-term consequences of childhood obesity are well documented and include elevated cardiovascular risk factors and respiratory comorbidities (Reilly, 2005). Less research has considered the long-term health impact of childhood obesity although it seems clear that many of the cardiovascular consequences that characterize adult-onset obesity are preceded by abnormalities that begin in childhood (Dietz, 1998).

Only a few studies provide information on long-term health effects associated with weight status in childhood and adolescence. In Table 2.2, 10 studies that examined the association between childhood weight status and adult morbidity and mortality are summarized. In most of the studies children or adolescents were included who were born in the period between 1920 and 1960. The most recent study conducted (The Cardiovascular Risk in Young Finns Study, Raitakari et al., 2003) included subjects born between 1962 and 1977. Overall, findings of the studies indicate that overweight children and adolescents have an increased risk of adverse levels of several coronary heart disease risk factors and various adult comorbidities such as cardiovascular diseases in adulthood (Mossberg, 1989; Must et al., 1992; Oren et al., 2003; Wright et al., 2001). Furthermore, a number of studies have suggested that the mortality risk in adulthood of subjects who were overweight or obese during childhood and adolescence is increased (Gunnell et al., 1998; Mossberg 1989; Must et al., 1992; Nieto, Szklo and Comstock, 1992). Freedman et al (2001) found that, after adjustment for adult weight, childhood weight status is not independently related to adult risk factor levels. In contrast, others have reported that the increased mortality and morbidity risk remained elevated after adjustment for adult weight (Gunnell et al., 1998; Lake, Power and Cole, 1997; Must et al., 1992; Oren et al., 2003).

Discussion

Tracking

In general, the literature on tracking shows that the association between childhood weight and adult weight strengthens with increasing age in childhood. However, prediction of adult obesity remains moderate. Wright et al. (2001), Trudeau et al. (2001) and Boreham et al. (2004) used two adiposity measures, BMI and skinfolds, and stronger correlations between childhood and adulthood were reported for BMI. These findings suggest that the association between childhood and adult BMI may mainly reflect tracking of body build, which is less subject to variation in adipose tissue than fatness. Another explanation may be that skinfolds have greater measurement error than height and weight. The child-to-adult tracking of BMI is stronger for subjects with obese parents. Since the prevalence of two obese parents is increasing, tracking is likely to strengthen in the next generation.

Health consequences

The available literature suggests an increased risk for all-cause mortality and cardiovascular mortality and several co-morbidities in adulthood from overweight and obesity during childhood. However, many of the studies also found that after adjusting for adult weight status most of the associations became weaker. This may reflect the influence of tracking of weight status rather than the relationship between childhood obesity and adult health. In cases of strong tracking, the relative contributions of adult and childhood weight status to the observed morbidity and mortality rates cannot be identified clearly. Although the studies reviewed suggest a relationship between childhood obesity and adult health, the nature of the relationship remains unclear as well as the underlying causes. In addition, it is difficult to ascertain what the best age is during the growing years to predict adult health status. The number of studies that can be used to base our assumptions on is still very small, thus more longitudinal data are needed.

Limitations

Reported results are dependent on the intervals between measurements, the length and age period of the follow-up, the measure of adiposity, cut-off points used to define overweight/obesity, and the ages used for prediction. A major shortcoming is that most studies have been performed in high-income countries. Outcomes may be quite different for populations in developing countries. Another limitation is that participants in most studies have grown up in very different circumstances from today's children. Therefore, data from these studies may not be representative of the tracking of the current generation.

Conclusion

We can conclude that the tracking of weight status from childhood to adulthood is moderate, and that childhood obesity is associated with several negative health consequences in adulthood. As correlations are not strong, future longitudinal studies are needed for more conclusive evidence.

Taking into consideration that the data of the longitudinal studies we described here are primarily based on cohort studies conducted more than 20 years ago, when prevalence of obesity was not as high as nowadays, the need for effective prevention in an early stage of life is even more compelling.

From a public health point of view we advise a population-based approach for the prevention of obesity, starting at an early age. Since tracking is stronger from adolescence to adulthood, and because risks of adult morbidity and mortality seem to be elevated for individuals who are overweight during adolescence, early adolescence seems an appropriate age period for promotion of healthy lifestyles.

References

Boreham, C., Robson, P.J., Gallagher, A.M., Cran, G.W., Savage, J.M. and Murray, L.J. (2004) 'Tracking of physical activity, fitness, body composition and diet from adolescence to young adulthood: the Young Hearts Project, Northern Ireland', *International Journal of Behavioral Nutrition and Physical Activity*, 1: 14.

Braddon, F.E., Rodgers, B., Wadsworth, M.E. and Davies, J.M. (1986) 'Onset of obesity in a 36 year birth cohort study', *British Medical Journal (Clinical Research Edition)*, 293: 299–303.

Casey, V.A., Dwyer, J.T., Coleman, K.A. and Valadian, I. (1992) 'Body mass index from childhood to middle age: a 50-y follow-up', *American Journal of Clinical Nutrition*, 56: 14–18.

Cole, T.J., Bellizzi, M.C., Flegal, K.M. and Dietz, W.H. (2000) 'Establishing a standard definition for child overweight and obesity worldwide: international survey', *British Medical Journal*, 320: 1240–3.

Deshmukh-Taskar, P., Nicklas, T.A., Morales, M., Yang, S.J., Zakeri, I. and Berenson, G.S. (2006) 'Tracking of overweight status from childhood to young adulthood: the Bogalusa Heart Study', *European Journal of Clinical Nutrition*, 60: 48–57.

Dietz, W.H. (1998) 'Health consequences of obesity in youth: childhood predictors of adult disease', *Pediatrics*, 101: 518–25.

Eriksson, J., Forsen, T., Tuomilehto, J., Osmond, C. and Barker, D. (2001) 'Size at birth, childhood growth and obesity in adult life', *International Journal of Obesity and Related Metabolic Disorders*, 25: 735–40.

Eriksson, J., Forsen, T., Osmond, C. and Barker, D. (2003) 'Obesity from cradle to grave', *International Journal of Obesity and Related Metabolic Disorders*, 27: 722–7.

Freedman, D.S., Khan, L.K., Dietz, W.H., Srinivasan, S.R. and Berenson, G.S. (2001), 'Relationship of childhood obesity to coronary heart disease risk factors in adulthood: the Bogalusa Heart Study', *Pediatrics*, 108: 712–18.

Gunnell, D.J., Frankel, S.J., Nanchahal, K., Peters, T.J. and Davey, S.G. (1998) 'Childhood obesity and adult cardiovascular mortality: a 57-y follow-up study based on the Boyd Orr cohort', *American Journal of Clinical Nutrition*, 67: 1111–18.

Guo, S.S., Roche, A.F., Chumlea, W.C., Gardner, J.D. and Siervogel, R.M. (1994) 'The predictive value of childhood body mass index values for overweight at age 35 years', *American Journal of Clinical Nutrition*, 59: 810–19.

Hulens, M., Beunen, G., Claessens, A.L., Lefevre, J., Thomis, M., Philippaerts, R., Borms, J., Vrijens, J., Lysens, R. and Vansant, G. (2001) 'Trends in BMI among Belgian children, adolescents and adults from 1969 to 1996', *International Journal of Obesity and Related Metabolic Disorders*, 25: 395–9.

Juonala, M., Raitakari, M., Viikari, S.A. and Raitakari, O.T. (2006) 'Obesity in youth is not an independent predictor of carotid IMT in adulthood. The Cardiovascular Risk in Young Finns Study', *Atherosclerosis*, 185: 388–93.

Kvaavik, E., Tell, G.S. and Klepp, K.I. (2003) 'Predictors and tracking of body mass index from adolescence into adulthood: follow-up of 18 to 20 years in the Oslo Youth Study', *Archives of Pediatric and Adolescent Medicine*, 157: 1212–18.

Laitinen, J., Power, C. and Jarvelin, M.R. (2001) 'Family social class, maternal body mass index, childhood body mass index, and age at menarche as predictors of adult obesity', *American Journal of Clinical Nutrition*, 74: 287–94.

Lake, J.K., Power, C. and Cole, T.J. (1997) 'Child to adult body mass index in the 1958 British birth cohort: associations with parental obesity, *Archive of Disease in Childhood*, 77: 376–81.

van Lenthe, F.J., Kemper, H.C., Van Mechelen, W. and Twisk, J.W. (1996) 'Development and tracking of central patterns of subcutaneous fat in adolescence and adulthood: the Amsterdam Growth and Health Study', *International Journal of Epidemiology*, 25: 1162–71.

Livingstone, M.B. (2001) 'Childhood obesity in Europe: a growing concern', *Public Health Nutrition*, 4: 109–16.

Magarey, A.M., Daniels, L.A., Boulton, T.J. and Cockington, R.A. (2003) 'Predicting obesity in early adulthood from childhood and parental obesity', *International Journal of Obesity and Related Metabolic Disorders*, 27: 505–13.

Martorell, R., Khan, L.K., Hughes, M.L. and Grummer-Strawn, L.M. (2000), 'Overweight and obesity in preschool children from developing countries', *International Journal of Obesity*, 24: 959–67.

Mossberg, H.O. (1989) '40-year follow-up of overweight children', *Lancet*, 2: 491–3.

Must, A. and Strauss, R.S. (1999) 'Risks and consequences of childhood and adolescent obesity'. *International Journal of Obesity and Related Metabolic Disorders*, 23(Suppl 2): S2–11.

Must, A., Jacques, P.F., Dallal, G.E., Bajema, C.J. and Dietz, W.H. (1992) 'Long-term morbidity and mortality of overweight adolescents. A follow-up of the Harvard Growth Study of 1922 to 1935', *New England Journal of Medicine*, 327: 1350–5.

Nieto, F.J., Szklo, M. and Comstock, G.W. (1992) 'Childhood weight and growth rate as predictors of adult mortality', *American Journal of Epidemiology*, 136: 201–13.

Oren, A., Vos, L.E., Uiterwaal, C.S., Gorissen, W.H., Grobbee, D.E. and Bots, M.L. (2003) 'Change in body mass index from adolescence to young adulthood and increased carotid intima-media thickness at 28 years of age: the Atherosclerosis Risk in Young Adults study', *International Journal of Obesity and Related Metabolic Disorders*, 27: 1383–90.

Peeters, A., Barendregt, J.J., Willekens, F., Mackenbach, J.P., Al Mamun, A., and Bonneux, I. (2003) 'Obesity in adulthood and its consequences for life expectancy: a life-table analysis', *Annals of Internal Medicine*, 138: 24–32.

Raitakari, O.T., Juonala, M., Kahonen, M., Taittonen, L., Laitinen, T., Maki-Torkko, N., Jarvisalo, M.J., Uhari, M., Jokinen, E., Ronnemaa, T., Akerblom, H.K. and Viikari, J.S. (2003) 'Cardiovascular risk factors in childhood and carotid artery intima-media thickness in adulthood: the Cardiovascular Risk in Young Finns Study', *Journal of the American Medical Association*, 290: 2277–83.

Reilly, J.J. (2005) 'Descriptive epidemiology and health consequences of childhood obesity', *Best Practice and Research Clinical Endocrinology Metabolism*, 19: 327–341.

Trudeau, F., Shephard, R.J., Arsenault, F. and Laurencelle, L. (2001) 'Changes in adiposity and body mass index from late childhood to adult life in the Trois-Rivieres Study', *American Journal of Human Biology*, 13: 349–55.

Twisk, J.W.R., Kemper, H.C.G. and Mellenbergh, G.J. (1994) 'Mathematical and analytical aspects of tracking', *Epidemiological Reviews*, 16: 165–83.

Twisk, J.W.R., Mechelen, W. and Kemper, H.C.G. (2000) 'Tracking of activity and fitness and the relationship with CVD risk factors', *Medicine Science in Sports and Exercise*, 32: 1455–61.

Vanhala, M., Vanhala, P., Kumpusalo, E., Halonen, P. and Takala, J. (1998) 'Relation between obesity from childhood to adulthood and the metabolic syndrome: population
based study', *British Medical Journal*, 317: 319.

Ware, J.H. and Wu, M.C. (1981) 'Tracking: prediction of future values from serial measurements', *Biometrics*, 37: 427–37.

Whitaker, R.C., Wright, J.A., Pepe, M.S., Seidel, K.D. and Dietz, W.H. (1997) 'Predicting
obesity in young adulthood from childhood and parental obesity', *New England Journal
of Medicine*, 337: 869–73.

Williams, S. (2001) 'Overweight at age 21: the association with body mass index in childhood and adolescence and parents' body mass index. A cohort study of New Zealanders
born in 1972–1973', *International Journal of Obesity and Related Metabolic Disorders*, 25:
158–63.

World Health Organization (1998) *Obesity, Preventing and Managing the Global Epidemic:
Report of the WHO Consultation of Obesity*, Geneva: World Health Organization.

Wright, C.M., Parker, L., Lamont, D. and Craft, A.W. (2001) 'Implications of childhood
obesity for adult health: findings from thousand families cohort study', *British Medical
Journal*, 323: 1280–8.

3 Clinical correlates of overweight and obesity

E. Denney-Wilson and L.A. Baur

Introduction

Obesity in childhood is not simply of cosmetic or even psychological concern; obese children and adolescents suffer co-morbidities affecting almost every body system. Immediate effects include social and psychological problems as well as significant medical morbidity, while long-term effects include the establishment of risk factors for cardiovascular disease and type 2 diabetes as well as the development of adult obesity.

The prevalence of complications

Although several studies have described otherwise rare conditions among clinical populations of severely obese children and adolescents, it is not known how the recent increases in the prevalence of obesity have affected the prevalence of obesity-associated complications amongst the general paediatric population. Most of the published studies have examined only one or two complications, rather than screening their cohort for the range of potential problems. Additionally, we do not know what levels of adiposity are associated with the range of complications; indeed, the associations between adiposity and complications may not be linear. Finally, the vast majority of overweight young people do not consider themselves unwell and do not seek consultation or treatment for their weight problem. We therefore cannot reliably estimate the true prevalence of complications without population-based studies. Table 3.1 summarizes the potential complications of obesity among children and adolescents.

As mentioned above, there are few estimates of the prevalence of obesity-associated complications. However, the rising prevalence of overweight and obesity in childhood and adolescence suggests that both the incidence and prevalence of obesity-associated complications are also increasing in this age group. Epidemiological evidence supports the theory that the association between obesity and disease risk begins early in life. For example, autopsies conducted on young adults who died from trauma found that fatty streaks in the coronary arteries and aorta were associated with blood lipid profile, blood pressure, and obesity measured at

Table 3.1 Potential obesity-associated complications among children and adolescents

System	Health problems
Psychosocial	Social isolation and discrimination, decreased self-esteem, learning difficulties, body image disorder, bulimia Medium- and long-term: Poorer social and economic 'success', bulimia
Respiratory	Obstructive sleep apnoea, asthma, poor exercise tolerance
Orthopaedic	Back pain, slipped femoral capital epiphyses, tibia vara, ankle sprains, flat feet
Gastrointestinal	Non-alcoholic fatty liver disease, gastro-oesophageal reflux and gastric emptying disturbances, gallstones
Reproductive	Polycystic ovary syndrome, menstrual abnormalities, infertility
Cardiovascular	Hypertension, adverse lipid profile (low HDL cholesterol, high triglycerides, high LDL cholesterol) Medium- and long-term: Increased risk of hypertension and adverse lipid profile in adulthood, increased risk of coronary artery disease in adulthood, left ventricular hypertrophy
Endocrine	Hyperinsulinaemia, insulin resistance, impaired glucose tolerance, impaired fasting glucose, type 2 diabetes mellitus Medium- and long-term: Increased risk of type 2 diabetes mellitus in adulthood
Neurological	Benign intracranial hypertension
Dermatological	Acanthosis nigricans, stretch marks, thrush

one or more points antemortem (Berenson *et al.*, 1998). Many obesity-related complications associated with childhood obesity take several years to develop although a number are immediately apparent. Although adverse health problems cannot be completely separated into time frames, for the purposes of this chapter complications will be reported by body system and as occurring in childhood and adolescence or in adulthood.

The importance of abdominal fat

Fat distribution is an important consideration when determining risk factors associated with obesity among young people as well as adults. Abdominal fat is more highly correlated with risk factors than total or per cent body fat (Daniels *et al.*, 1999; Maffeis *et al.*, 2001; Morrison *et al.*, 1999; Owens *et al.*, 2000) and is an independent risk factor for cardiovascular disease and type 2 diabetes (Goran and Gower, 1999). Among adults and children, the presence of high levels of abdominal fat is associated with the constellation of risk factors including hypertension, an adverse lipid profile, hyperinsulinaemia and glucose intolerance, known as the metabolic syndrome (Daniels *et al.*, 1999; Goran and Gower, 1999).

Complications occurring during childhood and adolescence

Immediate problems associated with obesity among young people include social exclusion and psychological dysfunction. In the short term, overweight children and adolescents may develop metabolic and orthopaedic problems and they may also have cardiovascular risk factors that could ultimately lead to long-term morbidity and mortality.

Psychological and social problems

Several studies have demonstrated psychological dysfunction and social isolation of overweight or obese children (Friedman *et al.*, 1995; Must and Strauss, 1999). At as early as six years of age, overweight children may be described by their peers as ugly, stupid, dishonest and lazy and as a result may experience teasing and social isolation (Hill and Silver 1995).

In adolescent girls, excess weight (as measured by body mass index [BMI]) is significantly related to body dissatisfaction, drive for thinness and bulimia as measured by the Eating Disorders Inventory (Friedman *et al.*, 1995). Cross-sectional studies of teenagers consistently show an inverse relationship between weight and both global self-esteem and body-esteem (French, Story and Perry, 1995). Adolescence is a period when there is marked self-awareness of body shape and physical appearance and so it is not surprising that the pervasive, negative social messages associated with obesity in many communities have an impact at this stage.

Respiratory problems

Respiratory outcomes can be poor in obese children. For example, 30 per cent of obese children have asthma, and, when compared with lean children with asthma, the overweight and obese children use more medications, have more wheezing episodes and experience more unscheduled visits to hospital (Belamarich *et al.*, 2000). Obese school-aged boys (but not girls), are almost three times more likely to have newly diagnosed asthma (Gilliland *et al.*, 2003). Obese children also have a lower exercise tolerance than their lean peers, perhaps compounding their obesity (Reybrouck *et al.*, 1997).

Potentially more serious is the complication of obstructive sleep apnoea. This is characterized by snoring, enlarged tonsils and adenoids, and periods of partial or complete airway obstruction while asleep, leading to recurrent hypoxia and sleep deprivation. A classic description of obstructive sleep apnoea is given in Charles Dickens' book *The Pickwick Papers*, published in 1837, in which Joe, 'the fat boy', is described as snoring and as being excessively sleepy during the day (Dickens, 1966).

Obstructive sleep apnoea may be associated with obesity, insulin resistance and dyslipidaemia among children and adolescents, and increases in severity in association with increased fasting insulin (de la Eva *et al.*, 2002). Children with sleep apnoea may suffer long-term consequences including hypertension and increased cardiovascular morbidity (Redline *et al.*, 1999). Profound hypoventilation and even sudden death have been reported in severe cases of sleep apnoea associated with obesity (Riley, Santiago and Edelman, 1976).

Orthopaedic problems

Orthopaedic complications are well recognized in obese children, and otherwise rare disorders occur with greater frequency among obese individuals. For example, in an international multi-centre study, 63 per cent of children with slipped capital femoral epiphyses had a body weight which was greater than or equal to the ninetieth percentile for age (Loder, 1996). In this problem, the femoral epiphysis is subjected to the increased stress of weight bearing, with eventual slippage occurring. Obesity may also be associated with the development of Blount's disease (tibia vara), in which there is a deformity of the medial portion of the proximal tibial metaphysis (Dietz, Gross and Kirkpatrick, 1982). This deformity arises as a result of increased, and possibly unconventional, weight bearing on cartilaginous bone with subsequent compensatory overgrowth and bowing of the tibia (Henderson and Greene, 1994). Young people who are overweight or obese have low bone area and bone mass relative to their body weight, making them more prone to fractures than lean individuals (Goulding *et al.*, 2000).

As well as serious forms of orthopaedic disease, more minor abnormalities are also seen, including knock knee (genu valgum) and an increased susceptibility to ankle sprains. Obese children have flat, wide feet with increased static and dynamic plantar pressures (Dowling, Steele and Baur, 2001); this may put them at risk of a range of minor orthopaedic problems. These conditions may seem relatively trivial in health terms, but have a significant impact on a child's quality of life and ability to participate fully in activities.

Gastrointestinal problems

Obese children and adolescents may experience gastrointestinal disorders including gallstones and non-alcoholic fatty liver disease (Must and Strauss, 1999). Obesity is the cause of 8–33 per cent of the cases of gallstones in children, and is the major cause in children without other medical problems. Non-alcoholic fatty liver disease is a common complication of obesity among children and adolescents, recent studies indicating a prevalence of 40–52 per cent among children and adolescents with severe obesity (Guzzaloni *et al.*, 2000). The disorder is characterized by elevated liver enzymes and in the long term may lead to liver fibrosis and cirrhosis. The only treatment for this condition is weight loss and treatment of the associated insulin resistance (Manton *et al.*, 2000).

Gastro-oesophageal reflux and gastric emptying disturbances are further complications of childhood obesity and appear to be a consequence of raised intra-abdominal pressure due to increased subcutaneous and visceral fat.

Reproductive complications

Menstrual abnormalities occur more frequently in obese girls, including the early onset of puberty and menarche, as well as menstrual irregularities and polycystic ovaries. There is a strong association between abdominal fat, increased levels of the androgenic hormones, hirsutism, insulin resistance and polycystic ovaries, which grouped together is termed polycystic ovary syndrome. Polycystic ovary syndrome is associated with infertility among adult women, with weight loss improving fertility outcomes (Homberg, 2003).

Cardiovascular problems

Risk factors for cardiovascular disease are one of the most common problems facing the obese young person. Data from the Bogalusa Heart Study in the United States indicate that 60 per cent of overweight 5- to 10-year-olds have one cardiovascular risk factor, such as hypertension, high LDL cholesterol, high triglycerides, while over 20 per cent had two or more risk factors (Freedman *et al.*, 1999). Overall, when compared with their lean peers overweight children are 2.4 times as likely to have elevated total cholesterol and diastolic blood pressure and 4.5 times as likely to have elevated systolic blood pressure. Similar findings were reported by Chu (2001) from the Taipei Children Heart study, who reported a significant association between obesity and higher blood pressure, blood glucose and blood lipids.

Endocrine problems

Although relatively rare among children and adolescents, the incidence of type 2 diabetes mellitus is increasing dramatically and is inextricably linked to the prevalence of obesity among young people. Clinical research from the United States has reported a tenfold increase in the incidence of type 2 diabetes among an adolescent population, from 0.7/100,000 per year in 1982, to 7.2/100,000 per year in 1994. All of the newly diagnosed adolescents were obese, and had a strong family history of type 2 diabetes (Pinhas-Hamicl *et al.*, 1996). Other research in the United States suggests that between 8 and 45 per cent of new cases of diabetes are of type 2 diabetes, with obesity, a sedentary lifestyle and genetic predisposition being major contributing factors to its development (Rocchini, 2002).

Type 2 diabetes does not occur suddenly; rather, it is a disorder that develops over a period of time and is characterized by gradual deterioration of the function of the pancreas. Initially, insulin resistance may be present, followed subsequently by impaired fasting glucose or glucose intolerance. Both impaired glucose tolerance and insulin resistance are more common in overweight and obese children and adolescents (Srinivasan, Myers and Berenson, 1999). Data from the Bogalusa Heart Study indicate that overweight children are 12.6 times more likely to have elevated fasting insulin concentrations than their lean peers (Freedman *et al.*, 1999).

The metabolic syndrome was initially identified among adults, but evidence has now emerged that abdominal fat among children is also highly correlated with risk factors such as elevated fasting insulin and lipid concentrations (Srinivasan, Myers and Berenson, 2002). The syndrome is defined as a constellation of risk factors including the presence of excess abdominal fat, hypertension, dyslipidaemia and insulin resistance. Among 12- to 19-year-olds in the United States, the prevalence of the metabolic syndrome is 4.2 per cent overall; however, among overweight adolescents, the metabolic syndrome affects 28.7 per cent of individuals (Cook *et al.*, 2003). Any further increases in the prevalence of obesity are likely to be accompanied by increases in the significant morbidity associated with this disorder.

Neurological problems

Benign intracranial hypertension, or pseudotumor cerebri, is a rare but very serious complication of obesity among children and adolescents (Must and Strauss, 1999). This disorder is characterized by severe headache, disturbed vision and vomiting caused by raised intracranial pressure (Zwiauer *et al.*, 2002).

Skin problems

Obese children suffer from overheating as their fat tissue acts as insulation, resulting in profuse sweating with any physical activity. Thrush occurs more commonly in obese subjects, especially in such moist, overheated areas as skinfolds or the groin. Stretch marks can also occur, particularly on the abdomen and thighs. A more serious complication, in terms of its being a marker of insulin resistance, is acanthosis nigricans, a condition characterized by thickened areas of pigmentation, particularly in skinfolds, the base of the neck, axillae and the groin. As with many orthopaedic problems, skin problems associated with obesity may seem relatively minor, but may cause substantial embarrassment to the obese young person.

Adult complications arising from child and adolescent obesity

The most significant health risk faced by obese young people is that they are highly likely to become obese adults, and therefore be at increased risk of cardiovascular disease, diabetes and some cancers. Tracking of weight status is related to the degree of overweight and the age of onset (Whitaker *et al.*, 1997). However, as the epidemic of obesity among children is a relatively recent phenomenon, studies to date examining the prevalence of tracking of weight status into adulthood were necessarily done in a population with a relatively lower prevalence of overweight during their childhood. As BMI in childhood is correlated with BMI in adulthood (Wattigney *et al.*, 1995), and both obesity-related behaviours and BMI track into adulthood (Berkey *et al.*, 2000), it is possible that an even greater proportion of the adult population will be overweight or obese in the future.

Psychosocial problems

Overweight in adolescence may also be associated with later social and economic problems. A large prospective study from the United States has shown that women who are overweight in late adolescence and early adulthood are more likely, as adults, to have lower family incomes, higher rates of poverty and lower rates of marriage than women with other forms of chronic physical disability but who were not overweight (Gortmaker *et al.*, 1993). These findings are likely to reflect the impact of social discrimination against obese persons.

Cardiovascular complications

Obesity in childhood and adolescence is associated with increased risk of heart disease in adulthood. For example, in a cohort in the United Kingdom followed up over a 57-year period, both all-cause and cardiovascular mortality were associated with higher childhood BMI (Gunnell *et al.*, 1998). Study participants who, as children were heavier than the seventy-fifth centile for BMI, were twice as likely to die from ischaemic heart disease as those who, as children, had a BMI between the twenty-fifth and seventy-fifth centiles. In a similar long-term (55-year) follow-up of a United States cohort of adolescents, overweight in adolescence was a significant predictor of morbidity and mortality from cardiovascular disease, independent of adult weight status (Must *et al.*, 1992).

Endocrine and metabolic complications

Individuals who were overweight as children have an increased risk of endocrine and metabolic complications as adults. Data from the Bogalusa Heart Study indicate that, by age 30, 2.4 per cent of those who had been overweight as children (defined as a BMI greater than the seventy-fifth centile) had developed type 2 diabetes, compared with none of the lean children (Freedman *et al.*, 1999).

Individuals with diabetes are at risk of serious co-morbidity. In the United States, diabetes is responsible for half of all non-traumatic amputations, 15 per cent of blindness and more than 30 per cent of all end-stage renal disease (Rao, 1999). Adolescents with type 2 diabetes often have poor glucose control which may precipitate early diabetic complications (Fagot-Campagna *et al.*, 2000). The early onset and increasing prevalence of this disease could pose a major public health problem as more people develop long-term complications at younger ages.

Data from a large cross-sectional study in the United States indicate that the metabolic syndrome affects over 20 per cent of 20- to 29-year-olds and over 40 per cent of adults aged 60–70 years (Ford, Giles and Dietz, 2002). Childhood obesity is a significant predictor of the metabolic syndrome among adults, with data from the Bogalusa Heart Study indicating that childhood BMI is the strongest predictor of the development of the cluster of risk factors that characterize the syndrome. The study found that those children who were in the top quartile of BMI were 11 times more likely to develop the metabolic syndrome as adults than their lean peers (Srinivasan, Myers and Berenson, 2002).

Conclusion

Obesity is a complex disorder with many associated complications. Even if an obese child achieves a healthy adult weight, they are still at risk of substantial morbidity. Evidence to date suggests that primary prevention and treatment focusing on children is needed to improve long-term population health outcomes. As the last decade has shown a dramatic increase in the prevalence of obesity among children and evidence of correlations between childhood obesity and cardiovascular disease and diabetes, major challenges await health professionals in the years to come.

References

Belamarich, P.F., Luder, E., Kattan, M., Mitchell, H., Islam, S., Lynn, H. and Crain, E.F. (2000) 'Do obese inner-city children with asthma have more symptoms than nonobese children with asthma?', *Pediatrics*, 106: 1436–42.

Berenson, G.S., Srinivasan, S.R., Bao, W., Newman, W.P. III, Tracy, R.E. and Wattigney, W.A. (1998) 'Association between multiple cardiovascular risk factors and atherosclerosis in children and young adults', *New England Journal of Medicine*, 338: 1650–6.

Berkey, C.S., Rockett, H.R., Field, A.E., Gillman, M.W., Frazier, A.L., Camargo, C.A. Jr and Colditz, G.A. (2000) 'Activity, dietary intake, and weight changes in a longitudinal study of preadolescent and adolescent boys and girls', *Pediatrics*, 105: E56.

Chu, N.F. (2001) 'Prevalence and trends of obesity among school children in Taiwan: the Taipei Children Heart Study', *International Journal of Obesity Related Metabolic Disorders*, 25: 170–6.

Cook, S., Weitzman, M., Auinger, P., Nguyen, M. and Dietz, W.H. (2003) 'Prevalence of a metabolic syndrome phenotype in adolescents: findings from the Third National Health and Nutrition Examination Survey, 1988–1994', *Archives of Pediatrics and Adolescent Medicine*, 157: 821–7.

Daniels, S.R., Morrison, J.A., Sprecher, D.L., Khoury, P. and Kimball, T.R. (1999) 'Association of body fat distribution and cardiovascular risk factors in children and adolescents', *Circulation*, 99: 541–5.

Dickens, C. (1966) *The Posthumous Papers of the Pickwick Club*, London: Oxford University Press.

Dietz, W.H., Jr, Gross, W.L. and Kirkpatrick, J.A., Jr (1982) 'Blount disease (tibia vara): another skeletal disorder associated with childhood obesity', *Journal of Pediatrics*, 101: 735–7.

Dowling, A.M., Steele, J.R. and Baur, L.A. (2001) 'Does obesity influence foot structure and plantar pressure patterns in prepubescent children?', *International Journal of Obesity Related Metabolic Disorders*, 25: 845–52.

de la Eva, R.C., Baur, L.A., Donaghue, K.C. and Waters, K.A. (2002) 'Metabolic correlates with obstructive sleep apnea in obese subjects', *Journal of Pediatrics*, 140: 654–9.

Fagot-Campagna, A., Pettitt, D.J., Engelgau, M.M., Burrows, N.R., Geiss, L.S., Valdez, R., Beckles, G.L., Saaddine, J., Gregg, E.W., Williamson, D.F. and Narayan, K.M. (2000) 'Type 2 diabetes among North American children and adolescents: an epidemiologic review and a public health perspective', *Journal of Pediatrics*, 136: 664–72.

Ford, E.S., Giles, W.H. and Dietz, W.H. (2002) 'Prevalence of the metabolic syndrome among US adults: findings from the Third National Health and Nutrition Examination Survey', *Journal of the American Medical Association*, 287: 356–9.

Freedman, D.S., Dietz, W.H., Srinivasan, S.R. and Berenson, G.S. (1999) 'The relation of overweight to cardiovascular risk factors among children and adolescents: the Bogalusa Heart Study', *Pediatrics*, 103: 82.

French, S.A., Story, M. and Perry, C.L. (1995) 'Self-esteem and obesity in children and adolescents: a literature review', *Obesity Research*, 3: 479–90.

Friedman, M.A., Wilfley, D.E., Pike, K.M., Striegel-Moore, R.H. and Rodin, J. (1995) 'The relationship between weight and psychological functioning among adolescent girls', *Obesity Research*, 3: 57–62.

Gilliland, F.D., Berhane, K., Islam, T., McConnell, R., Gauderman, W.J., Gilliland, S.S., Avol, E. and Peters, J.M. (2003) 'Obesity and the risk of newly diagnosed asthma in school-age children', *American Journal of Epidemiology*, 158: 406–15.

Goran, M.I. and Gower, B.A. (1999) 'Relation between visceral fat and disease risk in children and adolescents', *American Journal of Clinical Nutrition*, 70: S149–56.

Gortmaker, S.L., Must, A., Perrin, J.M., Sobol, A.M. and Dietz, W.H. (1993) 'Social and economic consequences of overweight in adolescence and young adulthood', *New England Journal of Medicine*, 329: 1008–12.

Goulding, A., Taylor, R.W., Jones, I.E., McAuley, K.A., Manning, P.J. and Williams, S.M. (2000) 'Overweight and obese children have low bone mass and area for their weight', *International Journal of Obesity Related Metabolic Disorders*, 24: 627–32.

Gunnell, D.J., Frankel, S.J., Nanchahal, K., Peters, T.J. and Davey, S.G. (1998) 'Childhood obesity and adult cardiovascular mortality: a 57-y follow-up study based on the Boyd Orr cohort', *American Journal of Clinical Nutrition*, 67: 1111–18.

Guzzaloni, G., Grugni, G., Minocci, A., Moro, D. and Morabito, F. (2000) 'Liver steatosis in juvenile obesity: correlations with lipid profile, hepatic biochemical parameters and glycemic and insulinemic responses to an oral glucose tolerance test', *International Journal of Obesity Related Metabolic Disorders*, 24: 772–6.

Henderson, R.C. and Greene, W.B. (1994) 'Etiology of late-onset tibia vara: Is varus alignment a prerequisite?', *Journal of Pediatric Orthopedics*, 14: 143–6.

Hill, A.J. and Silver, E.K. (1995) 'Fat, friendless and unhealthy: 9-year-old children's perception of body shape stereotypes', *International Journal of Obesity Related Metabolic Disorders*, 19: 423–30.

Homberg, R. (2003) 'The management of infertility associated with polycystic ovary syndrome', *Reproductive Biology and Endocrinology*, 1(1): 109.

Loder, R.T. (1996) 'The demographics of slipped capital femoral epiphysis. An international multicenter study', *Clinical Orthopaedics and Related Research*, 322: 8–27.

Maffeis, C., Pietrobelli, A., Grezzani, A., Provera, S. and Tato, L. (2001) 'Waist circumference and cardiovascular risk factors in prepubertal children', *Obesity Research*, 9: 179–87.

Manton, N.D., Lipsett, J., Moore, D.J., Davidson, G.P., Bourne, A.J. and Couper, R.T. (2000) 'Non-alcoholic steatohepatitis in children and adolescents', *Medical Journal of Australia*, 173: 476–9.

Morrison, J.A., Sprecher, D.L., Barton, B.A., Waclawiw, M.A. and Daniels, S.R. (1999) 'Overweight, fat patterning, and cardiovascular disease risk factors in black and white girls: the National Heart, Lung, and Blood Institute Growth and Health Study', *Journal of Pediatrics*, 135: 458–64.

Must, A. and Strauss, R.S. (1999) 'Risks and consequences of childhood and adolescent obesity', *International Journal of Obesity and Related Metabolic Disorders*, 23(Suppl 2): S2–11.

Must, A., Jacques, P.F., Dallal, G.E., Bajema, C.J. and Dietz, W.H. (1992) 'Long-term morbidity and mortality of overweight adolescents. A follow-up of the Harvard Growth Study of 1922 to 1935', *New England Journal of Medicine*, 327: 1350–5.

Owens, S., Gutin, B., Barbeau, P., Litaker, M., Allison, J., Humphries, M., Okuyama, T. and Le, N.A. (2000) 'Visceral adipose tissue and markers of the insulin resistance syndrome in obese black and white teenagers', *Obesity Research*, 8: 287–93.

Pinhas-Hamiel, O., Dolan, L.M., Daniels, S.R., Standiford, D., Khoury, P.R. and Zeitler, P. (1996) 'Increased incidence of non-insulin-dependent diabetes mellitus among adolescents', *Journal of Pediatrics*, 128: 608–15.

Rao, G. (1999) 'Diagnostic yield of screening for type 2 diabetes in high-risk patients: a systematic review', *Journal of Family Practice*, 48: 805–10.

Redline, S., Tishler, P.V., Schluchter, M., Aylor, J., Clark, K. and Graham, G. (1999) 'Risk factors for sleep-disordered breathing in children. Associations with obesity, race, and respiratory problems', *American Journal of Respiratory and Critical Care Medicine*, 159: 1527.

Reybrouck, T., Mertens, L., Schepers, D., Vinckx, J. and Gewillig, M. (1997) 'Assessment of cardiorespiratory exercise function in obese children and adolescents by body mass-independent parameters', *European Journal of Applied Physiology and Occupational Physiology*, 75: 478–83.

Riley, D.J., Santiago, T.V. and Edelman, N.H. (1976) 'Complications of obesity-hypoventilation syndrome in childhood', *American Journal of Diseases of Children*, 130: 671.

Rocchini, A.P. (2002) 'Childhood obesity and a diabetes epidemic', *New England Journal of Medicine*, 346: 854–5.

Srinivasan, S.R., Myers, L. and Berenson, G.S. (1999) 'Temporal association between obesity and hyperinsulinemia in children, adolescents, and young adults: the Bogalusa Heart Study', *Metabolism: Clinical and Experimental*, 48: 928–34.

Srinivasan, S.R., Myers, L. and Berenson, G.S. (2002) 'Predictability of childhood adiposity and insulin for developing insulin resistance syndrome (syndrome X) in young adulthood: the Bogalusa Heart Study', *Diabetes*, 51: 204–9.

Wattigney, W.A., Webber, L.S., Srinivasan, S.R. and Berenson, G.S. (1995) The emergence of clinically abnormal levels of cardiovascular disease risk factor variables among young adults: the Bogalusa Heart Study', *Preventative Medicine*, 24: 617–26.

Whitaker, R.C., Wright, J.A., Pepe, M.S., Seidel, K.D. and Dietz, W.H. (1997) 'Predicting obesity in young adulthood from childhood and parental obesity', *New England Journal of Medicine*, 337: 869–73.

Zwiauer, K., Caroli, M., Malecka-Tendera, E. and Poskitt, E. (2002) 'Clinical features, adverse effects and outcome', in W. Burniat, T.J. Cole, I. Lissau, E.M.E. Poskitt (eds) *Child and Adolescent Obesity*, Cambridge: Cambridge University Press, pp. 131–53.

Case history: Trudy, a 13-year-old girl with obesity

Trudy presented to her family doctor with a respiratory tract infection. During the consultation her mother commented that Trudy was concerned about her weight and that she was being teased at school. Indeed, she had left her previous school because of bullying and now it appeared to be starting afresh in the new school.

Trudy is the only child. She appears to have a good relationship with her parents and does have some good peer relationships. Her general health has been good, apart from the weight gain. Several family members are obese including her mother and three of her grandparents. In addition, her paternal grandfather has been recently diagnosed with type 2 diabetes and her maternal grandfather has hypercholesterolaemia and ischaemic heart disease.

Trudy leads a sedentary lifestyle, her main interests being playing music, sewing, reading and talking on the phone. She is driven to and from school each day and watches about 3 hours of television per day. Trudy's dietary intake includes such at-risk features as occasionally skipping breakfast, full cream milk, 'something nice' for morning and afternoon tea, regularly buying food at the milk-bar in the afternoon, having about 500 ml of soft drink per day and unlimited access to biscuits from the cupboards at home.

On examination, Trudy's height was 161.5 cm (< seventy-fifth centile), weight 74.3 kg (> ninety-seventh centile) and BMI 28.4 kg/m² (> ninety-fifth centile for age; adult overweight range). Her waist circumference was 89 cm (adult female 'at significant risk of metabolic complications' range). She was in mid-puberty and there were stretch marks on her abdomen and upper thighs. Her blood pressure was 120/80. A fasting blood test showed a normal glucose (4.6 mmol/L; normal range 3.5–5.5), hyperinsulinaemia (?17 pmol/L) and a lipid profile characteristic of central obesity. total cholesterol 5.3 mmol/L (normal range 2.6–5.5), HDL cholesterol 0.8 mmol/L (normal > 0.9), triglycerides 1.9 mmol/L (normal range 0.6–1.7).

Management

The family doctor arranged to see Trudy and her mother, both separately and together, initially every 3 weeks, and then less frequently. Two visits to a local dietician were also arranged, although there was a long waiting list and more frequent follow-up could not be organized. Trudy was encouraged to set her own goals for food and activity changes; these goals were revisited at the consultations. The whole family was supported to make changes to their eating patterns and the use of the television in the home. The dietician spent time with Trudy, looking at ways in which eating cues could be recognized and dealt with.

Progress

Over time, Trudy's mother herself started to lose weight as a result of altered cooking practices and being more active. Water was offered at the evening meal instead of a soft drink, less healthy snacks and biscuits were no longer stored in the cupboards and the whole family moved to eating more vegetables and having smaller meat portions at the evening meal. Trudy had at least something to eat for breakfast each morning and started walking to and from school each day. She started tennis lessons and found an interest in tap dancing.

Ten months later, Trudy's weight was 69.3 kg, height 163.0 cm, BMI 26.1 kg/m^2 and waist circumference 81 cm. She reported being fitter and said that she was greatly enjoying school and was no longer being bullied. A repeat fasting blood test showed an improved lipid profile (total cholesterol 4.8 mmol/L, HDL cholesterol 0.9 mmol/L, triglycerides 1.4 mmol/L) and a decreased insulin concentration (154 μmol/L), consistent with a reduction in central obesity.

4 Body composition assessment in children and adolescents – implications for obesity

A.P. Hills and M. Kagawa

Introduction

The two main anthropometric indicators of physical growth in children and adolescents are body height and weight. Routine assessment of height and weight in youngsters and comparison with normative data provide key information about physical maturation and nutritional status, including level of overweight. Similarly, such information provides a means of simple comparison between children of the same chronological age. One of the defining features of childhood obesity is early physical maturation (see Chapter 3). Earlier maturation of obese individuals is reflected in height and weight differences compared to normal weight youngsters. The ratio of height and weight, the body mass index (BMI), provides another means of categorizing level of overweight and physical status.

The aim of this chapter is to provide an overview of the main anthropometric and body composition techniques with relevance to overweight and obesity in youngsters. A concurrent aim is to address the relative merits of each of the techniques presented. However, the chapter is not intended to be a comprehensive appraisal of the area and readers are strongly encouraged to access key kinanthropometry (Norton and Olds, 2001) and body composition review material to source additional detail (Brodie, Moscrip and Hutcheon, 1998; Lobstein, Baur and Uauy, 2004; Wells and Fewtrell, 2006; Zemel, Riley and Stallings, 1997).

Changes in body composition

Growth and development during the childhood years is generally characterized as slow and gradual; however, marked changes in physical size, shape and body composition occur during puberty. During the adolescent period to follow, both genders show significant body weight increases with peak weight velocity in girls occurring approximately 6–9 months later than peak height velocity. In boys, peak height and weight velocity occur at approximately the same time. The preferential deposition of body fat in girls and skeletal muscle in boys are the defining body composition changes during the adolescent years. The combined effects of body fat increase and/or change in deposition, and skeletal changes result in the characteristic android and gynoid shape in males and females, respectively (Rogol, Clark and Roemmich, 2000).

Assessment of body composition

The assessment of body composition in children and adolescents is challenging because of differential maturation at a given chronological age. A number of publications provide a thorough overview of the assessment of body composition in pediatric populations and the reader is encouraged to source this material (Brodie, Moscrip and Hutcheon, 1997; Claessens, Beunen and Malina, 2000; Ellis, 2004; Goran, 1998; Heyward, 1998; Heyward and Wagner, 2004; Hills, Lyell and Byrne, 2001; Parker *et al.*, 2003; Pietrobelli, Peroni and Faith, 2003; Zemel, Riley and Stallings, 1997).

Body composition assessment methods at best provide estimations or predictions. Therefore all methods except cadaver analyses are described as indirect. More exactly, many techniques should be described as doubly indirect if they build on the measurements and assumptions of another indirect method and the inherent estimation errors (Hills and Parízková, 2002; Hills, Byrne and Parízková, 1998).

The most common approach to body composition analysis is to subdivide the body mass (weight) into two or more compartments based on elemental, chemical, anatomical or fluid components (Heymsfield and Masako, 1991; Wang *et al.*, 1993). The indirect assessment of body composition has routinely used the two-compartment model, that is to divide the body into fat mass (FM) and fat-free mass (FFM). However, advances in chemical and isotope-based methods have enabled further subdivision of the FFM into water, mineral and protein; in addition, imaging techniques have enabled the consideration of body composition in terms of fat, muscle, bone and other soft tissue (Brodie, Moscrip and Hutcheon, 1997; Heymsfield *et al.*, 2005; Roemmich *et al.*, 1997; Wells *et al.*, 1999).

Two of the inherent assumptions in the two-compartment model are:

- the constant densities of FM and FFM (0.9 g/mL and 1.1 g/mL, respectively) (Visser *et al.*, 1997);
- the relative amounts of the three major components of the FFM (aqueous, mineral and protein) are known, additive, and constant in all individuals (Classey *et al.*, 1999).

As a consequence, when the two-compartment model is used with children and adolescents who differ from the reference population in bone mineralization or hydration of FFM, the model has serious limitations. The chemical composition of the FFM does not reach adult values until approximately 17–20 years of age. As a result, the FM is commonly overestimated in children and adolescents when the two-compartment model is employed (Reilly, 1998).

The range of available body composition assessment methods is extensive. The extremes range from relatively simple and inexpensive field methods to more complex and expensive laboratory techniques requiring advanced equipment. An understanding of the relative merits of each approach or the strengths and weaknesses of each is essential. Such an understanding is important in choosing the best method to match the particular needs or requirements for body composition information (Durnin, 1995; Hills and Parízková, 2002).

The most field methods include anthropometric measures such as height, weight, skinfolds and circumferences, and the portable and relatively simple bioelectrical impedance analysis (BIA) approach. The more expensive laboratory methods include hydrodensitometry, air plethysmography (Pea Pod and Bod Pod™), dual energy X-ray absorptiometry (DXA), total body water (TBW) measurement, magnetic resonance imaging (MRI), computerized tomography (CT) and total body potassium (TBK). These body composition methodologies are generally not available to most researchers and therefore are out of the reach of most school teachers, coaches, and exercise and sport scientists.

Anthropometry

Anthropometric measures include height and weight, body proportions, circumference or girth measures, skinfold thickness, skeletal diameters, and segment lengths (Hills, Lyell and Byrne, 2001). Measures of relative fatness include weight and weight-for-height, circumferences (most commonly waist and hip), skinfold thickness and indices derived from height and weight measures. The most widely used index of relative fatness is the body mass index (BMI) (Cole, 2002; Cole *et al.*, 2005; Lobstein, Baur and Uauy, 2004; McCarthy *et al.*, 2006). The major advantages of anthropometric techniques are that they are generally non-invasive and equipment is commonly portable and therefore suited to use in a wide range of settings. Perhaps most importantly, anthropometry is often the preferred approach because it is relatively inexpensive. Despite the apparent simplicity of the approach, it is important to appreciate that the usefulness of anthropometric measurements is very much dependent upon the experience and reliability of the measurer (Ogle *et al.*, 1995).

Body mass index (BMI)

Despite BMI (weight [kg]/height squared [m^2]) being the most common anthropometric index to predict relative overweight (Hall and Cole, 2006), the appropriateness of the index in children and adolescents has been questioned. BMI does not measure body fatness per se and therefore may not be sensitive to differences in actual body composition, including the influence of race. In youngsters less than 15 years of age, BMI is not totally independent of height, and individuals with the same BMI may be quite different in terms of proportion of body fat and skeletal muscle tissue. Prediction of body composition from BMI may therefore be more reliable in individuals within the normal range for body weight and BMI, and biased in individuals with high or low body fat content. Two of the widely used Centers for Disease Control (CDC) BMI-for-age charts (Figures 4.1 and 4.2) are

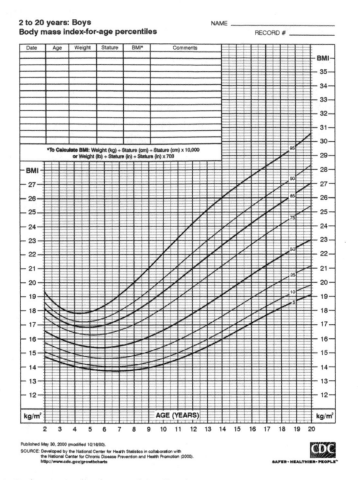

Figure 4.1 Body mass index-for-age chart (boys).

outlined in this chapter along with the compilation table by Cole *et al.* (2000) that provides cut-off values for overweight and obesity up to 18 years of age (Table 4.1). Readers are referred to the CDC website (http://www.cdc.gov/growthcharts).

Waist circumference

As a single measure, waist circumference is valued for its relationship with central adiposity in adults. The measure has gained increasing acceptance in younger people; however, cut-off points are not available to relate waist circumference to health status in children and adolescents (Rudolf *et al.*, 2004). The simple waist circumference measurement may be derived from one of three different measurement approaches. The preferred descriptor in this chapter is consistent with the definition of the International Society for the Advancement of Kinanthropometry (ISAK) and is the 'abdomen at its narrowest point between the lower costal (10th

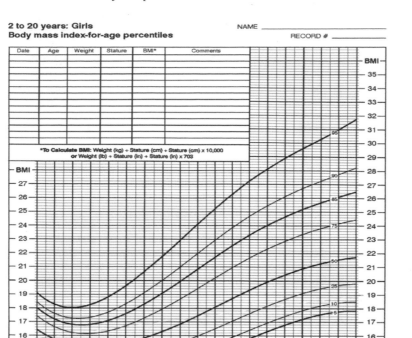

Figure 4.2 Body mass index-for-age chart (girls).

rib) border and the top of the iliac crest, perpendicular to the long axis of the trunk' (Marfell-Jones *et al.*, 2006). Readers are also encouraged to consult the book by Norton and Olds (2001) for more definitive information regarding this and other anthropometric measurements. The hip circumference (maximum girth of the hips and buttocks) and additional girth measurements may be used to profile the size and shape of individuals (Hills, Lyell and Byrne, 2001); however, the once commonly employed waist-to-hip ratio is no longer in vogue.

Skinfold thickness

Skinfold thickness measures have been used traditionally to assess the subcutaneous fat layer at multiple sites (Durnin and Womersley, 1974; Hills and Parízková, 2002). The double fold of skin and the underlying subcutaneous fat is measured using skinfold calipers (Hills, Lyell and Byrne, 2001).

Table 4.1 Cut-off values for overweight and obesity up to 18 years of age

Age (years)	Body mass index 25 kg/m²		Body mass index 30 kg/m²	
	Males	Females	Males	Females
2	18.41	18.02	20.09	19.81
2.5	18.13	17.76	19.80	19.55
3	17.89	17.56	19.57	19.36
3.5	17.69	17.40	19.39	19.23
4	17.55	17.28	19.29	19.15
4.5	17.47	17.19	19.26	19.12
5	17.42	17.15	19.30	19.17
5.5	17.45	17.20	19.47	19.34
6	17.55	17.34	19.78	19.65
6.5	17.71	17.53	20.23	20.08
7	17.92	17.75	20.63	20.51
7.5	18.16	18.03	21.09	21.01
8	18.44	18.35	21.60	21.57
8.5	18.76	18.69	22.17	22.18
9	19.10	19.07	22.77	22.81
9.5	19.46	19.45	23.39	23.46
10	19.84	19.86	24.00	24.11
10.5	20.20	20.29	24.57	24.77
11	20.55	20.74	25.10	25.42
11.5	20.89	21.20	25.58	26.05
12	21.22	21.68	26.02	26.67
12.5	21.56	22.14	26.43	27.24
13	21.91	22.58	26.84	27.76
13.5	22.27	22.98	27.25	28.20
14	22.62	23.34	27.63	28.57
14.5	22.96	23.66	27.98	28.87
15	23.29	23.94	28.30	29.11
15.5	23.60	24.17	28.60	29.29
16	23.90	24.37	28.88	29.43
16.5	24.19	24.54	29.14	29.56
17	24.46	24.70	29.41	29.69
17.5	24.73	24.85	29.70	29.84
18	25	25	30	30

The skinfold technique has the advantage of being reasonably inexpensive and able to be used in a wide range of settings due to the portability of equipment. Despite the sensitivity of some skinfold sites for some individuals, there is commonly a relatively low respondent burden for the most common sites. Despite the apparent simplicity of the skinfold technique, the approach does require a high degree of technical skill (Hills, Lyell and Byrne, 2001). As is the case for all anthropometric measures, reliability can be enhanced with quality training and experience including the use of standardized methods (see Norton and Olds, 2001, for comprehensive methodology). Unfortunately, measurement error is also related to the level of obesity of the individual being assessed such that skinfold measurements are notoriously unreliable in the obese. It is common for the skinfold thickness of an obese individual to exceed the maximum aperture of the caliper.

Perhaps thanks to the high level of interest in body fatness in the wider community, many people have been preoccupied with the conversion of skinfold measurements into a percentage body fat value. The conversion of raw skinfold data is an unnecessary step as satisfactory intra- and inter-individual comparisons can be made using the sum of skin fold measurements from representative sites. However, some research has suggested that equations using skinfolds are valid for use in young people (Durnin, 1995). The use of equations to derive total body fat values from skinfold measurements requires that one understands the potential impact of the changing relationship between subcutaneous fat (skinfolds) and total body fat during puberty and adolescence (Hills and Parízková, 2002).

Densitometry

Densitometry refers to the measurement of total body density and the estimation of body composition from body density. For many years, densitometry has been the mainstay in body composition assessment. Body density is the ratio of body mass to body volume, the latter measured by either water displacement or air displacement. Based on the assumed density constants of fat (0.9 g/mL) and FFM (1.1 g/mL) mentioned above and the measured density of the body, estimates of percentage body fat, FM and FFM can be derived using conversion formulae. For many years the hydrostatic (underwater weighing) technique was considered the 'gold standard' assessment method. Hydrostatic weighing is based on Archimedes' principle that the weight of the submerged individual is directly related to their body density (Hills, Lyell and Byrne, 2001) with body density representing a combination of the density of body fat and FFM. As for other approaches, there are a number of shortcomings with the underwater weighing technique in children, mainly due to the need for the child to submerge by exhaling air and then holding their breath for a number of seconds. Additional shortcomings of the approach relate to the key assumptions associated with the method. The underwater weighing technique assumes a constancy of the density of FFM; however, this is influenced by both hydration status and the contribution of BM to FFM (Lukaski, 1997). Each component is variable during the growing years and also dependent on diet and physical fitness.

Air-displacement plethysmography (Bod Pod™) represents a more suitable alternative to underwater weighing (Elia and Ward, 1999; Ellis *et al.*, 2007). However, a potential source of measurement error in both underwater weighing and air-displacement plethysmography is the conversion formula used to estimate per cent body fat from body density. Although densitometry yields an accurate measure of body density, some have speculated (Lohman, 1992) that variability in the FFM may lead to an error of approximately 2.8 per cent body fat when estimating relative body fat from body density in individuals of similar age, gender and ethnicity. As a result densitometry techniques are not considered the 'gold standard'.

Isotope dilution methods

The stable isotopes deuterium oxide (^2H_2O) and ^{18}O occur naturally in the body. The use of these isotopes is non-invasive, safe and effective in estimating total body water (TBW) in infants, children and adults (Wells *et al.*, 2005). Isotope dilution is used to estimate FFM and FM but, like underwater weighing, estimations assume a constant relationship between TBW and FFM and therefore fail to account for the chemical immaturity of the child. The hydration of lean FFM can vary before and after puberty.

Absorptiometry

Dual energy X-ray absorptiometry (DXA)

Total and regional body composition can be assessed using the DXA procedure. The method is based on the three-compartment model that divides the body into FM, bone mineral mass and lean body mass and is measured by attenuation of the dual energy X-ray beams. As each tissue varies in density, attenuation properties differ and this enables the determination of each of the tissue compartments. The precision of DXA in the measurement of percentage body fat is estimated as approximately 1.2 per cent body fat (Lohman, 1996). Further, DXA is highly reliable with good agreement between body fat estimates from underwater weighing and DXA. The radiation exposure from a DXA scan is extremely low and the procedure is quite fast so the technique has gained widespread acceptance for use in all age groups (particularly as an alternative to densitometry).

The advantages of the DXA technique may be summarized as follows (Heyward and Stolarczyk, 1996): it is highly reliable; measurement is rapid; minimal subject cooperation is required; and it accounts for differences in bone mineral density of subjects. Some of the main disadvantages include the requirement of further validation of the technique for children and also the ethical issues associated with exposure to radiation, albeit minimal. Heyward (1998) has indicated that estimates of FM depend on the manufacturer of the DXA equipment (i.e. Lunar, Hologic or Norland), the mode of data collection (pencil beam versus array beam) (Lohman, 1996) and the software used.

Hydrometry

Deuterium oxide dilution and bioelectrical impedance analysis (BIA)

The measurement of TBW or hydrometry also has limitations if used alone to generate reference measures of body composition. The use of the stable isotope deuterium oxide (^2H_2O) to estimate TBW is commonly recognized as the 'gold standard' (Wells *et al.*, 2003).

Bioelectrical impedance is an indirect method of measuring TBW. The BIA method involves passing a low-level electrical current through the body and measuring the impedance or opposition to the flow of current. The electrolytes in the body water are excellent conductors of electricity. Using an equation (different for each instrument), TBW and therefore FFM are calculated and FM (and usually percentage body fat) derived. Because adipose tissue is a relatively poor conductor of electricity on account of its small water content, the resistance in an individual with large amounts of body fat will be higher than that of an individual with a greater percentage of FFM. More recent research has considered measurement across multiple frequencies (MFBIA) instead of the customary single frequency and also segmental versus whole-body bioimpedance. The limbs primarily influence electrical resistance, which suggests that the BIA technique may be relatively insensitive to differences in tissue composition of the trunk (Zhu *et al.*, 1997).

Schaefer *et al.* (1994) found higher intra-observer and inter-observer reliability with BIA than with skinfold measures in youngsters with a mean age of 11.8 years; however, FFM estimates were similar for both BIA and anthropometry. Okasora *et al.* (1999) compared BIA and DXA as methods of body composition assessment in children and found close correlation between percentage BF, FFM and body fat content. The limitation of this study was that equations used by the researchers were those of Brozek *et al.* (1963). These equations are widely recognized as inappropriate for use in youth, as they do not account for the variability of the composition of the FFM in young individuals. Bland and Altman (1986) plots or an analysis of the size of the prediction error should be utilized to determine if there is agreement between the two measures.

The BIA technique is recognized as a useful body composition assessment technique in children and adolescents because measurement is fast and non-invasive. It is also inexpensive and painless, requires little subject cooperation, and does not require a high level of technical skill (Schaefer *et al.*, 1994). However the derived values using the BIA technique are only as good as the prediction equation utilized in the software. That is, if the group of individuals being assessed is representative of the population from whom the algorithm was derived the greater the potential value of the approach (Hills, Lyell and Byrne, 2001). The equations of Houtkeeper *et al.* (1992) are recommended for boys and girls 10–19 years of age. Further, the reliability of a method is dependent on the protocol used in the measurement. The following factors can influence BIA measurements: the level of hydration of the subject, posture, environmental and/or skin temperature, age, gender, athletic status, body composition status and ethnic origin. Ideally, if the BIA technique is used to assess changes in an individual over time, biological and environmental variables such as hydration status, timing and content of last ingested meal, skin temperature and menstrual cycle must be controlled for (Hills and Byrne, 1997; Jebb *et al.*, 2000).

Conclusions

BIA, skinfolds and anthropometry are the most appropriate for use in the field. These techniques are most commonly used at present as they have satisfactory validity provided that appropriate equations are used for the specific population (gender, age category, level of adaptation to exercise and so on). Useful prediction equations have been noted in this paper. BIA may hold the advantage over skinfolds as the technique is less invasive, requires less technical skill, has both higher inter-tester and intra-tester reliability, is quicker and may be easier to administer to a wider range of individuals. When experimental assessment is required, densitometry or DXA measurement procedures are preferred. This is especially the case when longitudinal observations are made (especially during puberty).

The three reference methods – densitometry, DXA and hydrometry – yield indirect estimates of body composition so none can be considered as the 'gold standard' for in vivo body composition assessment. Ideally for research purposes, the use of three methods is recommended in conjunction with a multi-component model to derive valid reference measurements of percentage body fat, FM and FFM (Heyward, 1998). Further development of methods for the evaluation of body composition is essential.

References

Bland, J.M. and Altman, D.G. (1986) 'Statistical methods for assessing agreement between two methods of clinical measurement', *Lancet*, 1: 307–10.

Brodie, D., Moscrip, V. and Hutcheon, R. (1998) 'Body composition measurement: a review of hydrodensitometry, anthropometry, and impedance methods', *Nutrition*, 14(3): 296–310.

Brozek, J., Grande, F., Anderson, J.T. and Keys, A. (1963) 'Densitometric analysis of body composition: revision of some quantitative assumptions', *Annals of the New York Academy of Sciences*, 110: 113–40.

Claessens, A.L., Beunen, G. and Malina, R.M. (2000) 'Anthropometry, physical and body composition and maturity', in N. Armstrong and W. van Mechelen (eds) *Paediatric Exercise Science and Medicine*, Oxford: Oxford University Press, pp. 11–22.

Classey, J.L., Kanaley, J.A., Wideman, L., Heymsfield, S.B., Teates, C.D., Gutgesell, M.E., Thorner, M.O., Hartman, M.L. and Weltman, A. (1999) 'Validity of methods of body composition assessment in young and older men and women', *Journal of Applied Physiology*, 86: 1728.

Cole, T.J. (2002) 'A chart to link child centiles of body mass index, weight and height', *European Journal of Clinical Nutrition*, 56(12): 1194–9.

Cole, T.J., Bellizzi, M.C., Flegal, K.M. and Dietz, W.H. (2000) 'Establishing a standard definition for child overweight and obesity worldwide: international survey', *British Medical Journal*, 320: 1240–3.

Cole, T.J., Faith, M.S., Pietrobelli, A. and Heo, M. (2005) 'What is the best measure of adiposity change in growing children: BMI, BMI%, BMI z-score or BMI centile?', *European Journal of Clinical Nutrition*, 59(3): 419–25.

Durnin, J.V.G.A. (1995) 'Appropriate technology in body composition: a brief review', *Asia Pacific Journal of Clinical Nutrition*, 4: 1.

Durnin, J.V.G.A. and Womersley, J. (1974) 'Body fat assessed from total body density and its estimation from skinfold thickness: measurements on 481 men and women aged from 16–72 years', *British Journal of Nutrition*, 32: 77.

Elia, M. and Ward, L.C. (1999) 'New techniques in nutritional assessment: body composition methods', *Proceedings of the Nutrition Society*, 58: 33.

Ellis, K.J. (2004) 'Body composition measurements', in W. Kiess, C. Marcus, M. Wabitsch (eds) *Obesity in Childhood and Adolescence. Pediatric and Adolescent Medicine*, Basel: Karger, vol. 9, pp. 20–9.

Ellis, K.J., Yao, M., Shypailo, R.J., Urlando, A., Wong, W.W. and Heird, W.C. (2007) 'Body composition assessment in infancy: air displacement plethysmogaphy compared with a reference 4-compartment model', *American Journal of Clinical Nutrition*, 85: 90–5.

Goran, M. (1998) 'Measurement issues related to studies of childhood obesity: assessment of body composition, body fat distribution, physical activity and food intake', *Pediatrics*, 101: 505–18.

Hall, D.M. and Cole, T.J. (2006) 'What use is the BMI?', *Archives of Diseases in Childhood*, 91(4): 283–6.

Heymsfield, S.B. and Masako, W. (1991) 'Body composition in humans: advances in the development of multicompartment chemical models', *Nutrition Reviews*, 49: 97.

Heymsfield S.B., Lohman, T., Wang, Z. and Going, S.B. (eds) (2005) *Human Body Composition*, Champaign, IL: Human Kinetics.

Heyward, V.H. (1998) 'Practical body composition assessment for children, adults, and older adults', *International Journal of Sports Nutrition*, 8(3): 285–307.

Heyward, V.H. and Stolarczyk, L.M. (1996) *Applied Body Composition Assessment*, Champaign, IL: Human Kinetics.

Heyward, V.H. and Wagner, D.H. (2004) *Applied Body Composition Assessment*, 2nd edition, Champaign, IL: Human Kinetics.

Hills, A.P. and Byrne, N.M. (1997) 'Bioelectrical impedance: use and abuse', in Coetsee, M.F., Van Heerden, H.J. (eds) *Proceedings of the International Council for Physical Activity and Fitness Research*, Itala: University of Zululand, p. 23.

Hills, A.P. and Parízková, J. (2002) 'Assessment of growth in adolescent athletes', in J.A. Driskell and I. Wolinsky (eds) *Nutritional Assessment of Athletes*, Boca Raton, FL: CRC Press.

Hills, A.P., Byrne, N.M. and Parízková, J. (1998) 'Methodological considerations in the assessment of physical activity and nutritional status of children and youth', in J. Parízková and A.P. Hills (eds) *Physical Fitness and Nutrition During Growth*, Basel: Karger, pp. 155–60.

Hills, A.P., Lyell, L. and Byrne, N.M. (2001) 'An evaluation of the methodology for the assessment of body composition in children and adolescents', in T. Jurimae and A.P. Hills (eds) *Body Composition Assessment in Children and Adolescents*, Basel: Karger.

Houtkeeper, L.B., Going, S.B., Lohman, T.G., Roche, A.F. and Van Loan, M. (1992) 'Bioelectrical impedance estimation of fat-free body mass in children and youth: a cross-validation study', *Journal of Applied Physiology*, 72: 366.

Jebb, S.A., Cole, T.J., Doman, D., Murgatroyd, P.R. and Prentice, A.M. (2000) 'Evaluation of the novel Tanita body-fat analyser to measure body composition by comparison with a four-compartment model', *British Journal of Nutrition*, 83(2): 115–22.

Lobstein, T., Baur, L. and Uauy, R. (2004) 'Obesity in children and young people: a crisis in public health', *Obesity Reviews*, 5(1): 4–85.

Lohman, T.G., (1992) *Advances in Body Composition Assessment*, Champaign, IL: Human Kinetics.

Lohman T.G. (1996) 'Dual energy X-ray absorptiometry', in Roche, A.F., Heymsfield, S.B., Lohman, T.G. (eds) *Human Body Composition*, Champaign, IL: Human Kinetics, pp. 63–78.

Lukaski, H.C. (1997) 'Methods for the assessment of human body composition: traditional and new', *American Journal of Clinical Nutrition*, 46: 537.

McCarthy, H.D., Cole, T.J., Fry, T., Jebb, S.A. and Prentice, A.M. (2006) 'Body fat reference curves for children', *International Journal of Obesity*, 30(4): 598–602.

Marfell-Jones, M., Olds, T., Stewart, A. and Carter, J.E.L. (2006) *International Standards for Anthropometric Assessment*, 2nd edition, Adelaide: The International Society for the Advancement of Kinanthropometry.

Norton, K. and Olds, T. (2001) *Anthropometrica*, Sydney: University of New South Wales Press.

Ogle, G.D., Allen, J.R., Humphries, I.R.J., Lu, P.W., Briody, J.N., Morely, K., Howman-Giles, R. and Cowell, C.T. (1995) 'Body composition assessment by dual energy x-ray absorptiometry in subjects aged 4–26 years', *American Journal of Clinical Nutrition*, 61: 746.

Okasora, K., Takaya, R., Tokuda, M., Fukunaga, Y., Oguni, T., Tanaka, H., Konishi, K. and Tamai, H. (1999) 'Comparison of bioelectrical impedance analysis and dual energy x-ray absorptiometry for assessment of body composition in children', *Pediatrics International*, 41: 121.

Parker, L., Reilly, J.J., Slater, C., Wells, J.C.K. and Pitsiladis, Y. (2003) 'Validity of six field and laboratory methods for measurement of body composition in boys', *Obesity Research*, 11: 852–8.

Pietrobelli, A., Peroni, D.G. and Faith, M.S. (2003) 'Pediatric body composition in clinical studies: which methods in which situations?', *Acta Diabetiologica*, 40: S270–3.

Reilly, J.J. (1998) 'Assessment of body composition in infants and children', *Nutrition*, 14: 821.

Roemmich, J.N., Clark, P.A., Weltman, A. and Rogol, A.D. (1997) 'Alterations in growth and body composition during puberty. I. Comparing multi-compartment body composition models', *Journal of Applied Physiology*, 83: 927.

Rogol, A.D., Clark, P.A. and Roemmich, J.N. (2000) 'Growth and pubertal development in children and adolescents: effects of diet and physical activity', *American Journal of Clinical Nutrition*, 72: 5215.

Rudolf, M.C., Greenwood, D.C., Cole, T.J., Levine, R., Sahota, P., Walker, J., Holland, P., Cade, J. and Truscott, J. (2004) 'Rising obesity and expanding waistlines in schoolchildren: a cohort study', *Archives of Diseases in Childhood*, 89(3): 235–7.

Schaefer, F., Georgi, M., Zieger, A. and Scharer, K. (1994) 'Usefulness of bioelectric impedance and skinfold measurements in predicting fat-free mass derived from total body potassium in children', *Pediatric Research*, 35: 617.

Slaughter, M.H., Lohman, T.G., Boileau, R.A., Horswill, C.A., Stillman, R.J., Van Loan, M.D. and Bemben, D.A. (1998) 'Skinfold equations for estimation of body fatness in children and youth', *Human Biology*, 60: 709.

Visser, M., Gallagher, D., Deurenberg, P., Wang, J., Pierson, R.N. and Heymsfield, S.B. (1997) 'Density and fat-free body mass: relationship with race, age, and level of fatness', *American Journal of Physiology*, 272: E781.

Wang, Z., Ma, R., Pierson, R.N. and Heymsfield, S.B. (1993) 'Five-level model: reconstruction of body weight at atomic, molecular, cellular, and tissue-system levels from neutron activation analysis', *Basic Life Sciences*, 60, 125.

Wells, J.C. and Fewtrell, M.S. (2006) 'Measuring body composition', *Archives of Diseases in Children*, 91: 612–17.

Wells, J.C.K., Fuller, N.J., Dewit, O., Fewtrell, M.S., Elia, M. and Cole, T.J. (1999) 'Four-compartment model of body composition in children: density and hydration of fat-free mass and comparison with simpler models', *American Journal of Clinical Nutrition*, 69, 904.

Wells, J.C., Fuller, N.J., Wright, A., Fewtrell, M.S. and Cole, T.J. (2003) 'Evaluation of air-displacement plethysmography in children aged 5–7 years using a three-component model of body composition', *British Journal of Nutrition*, 90(3): 485–6.

Wells, J.C., Fewtrell, M.S., Davies, P.S.W., Williams, J.E., Coward, W.A. and Cole, T.J. (2005) 'Prediction of total body water in infants and children', *Archives of Diseases in Children*, 90(9): 965–71.

Zemel, B.S., Riley, E.M. and Stallings, V.A. (1997) 'Evaluation of methodology for nutritional assessment in children: anthropometry, body composition and energy expenditure', *Annual Reviews of Nutrition*, 17: 211.

Zhu, F., Schneditz, D., Wang, E. and Levin, N.W. (1997) 'Dynamics of segmental extracellular volumes during changes in body position by bioelectrical impedance', *Journal of Applied Physiology*, 85: 497.

5 The importance of physical activity in the growth and development of children

N.M. Byrne and A.P. Hills

Introduction

Physical activity should be an integral part of normal growth and development for all young people. Early in life, particularly in infancy and early childhood, physical activity has an important role in the physical, psychosocial and mental development of the child. Most importantly, self-initiated informal play should be stressed, as the opportunity for the young child to experience a wide range of physical activities is likely to provide the greatest chance of developing the set of motor skills needed for participation in later lifestyle and/or sports activities.

The commonly cited health benefits of physical activity for young people include the prevention of overweight and obesity; improvement in skeletal health; enhancement of heart and lung function; and better psychological health. An ideal scenario for all youngsters would be the establishment of healthy lifestyle practices at a young age and the 'tracking' of regular physical activity participation into adulthood.

Despite the fact that chronic diseases such as obesity, cardiovascular disease, type 2 diabetes and osteoporosis are commonly identified as adult health problems, all have their genesis in the paediatric years. Another consistent feature of each chronic disease is the potential for physical activity to play a central role in effective prevention, treatment and management. In short, in combination with sound nutritional practices, adequate physical activity represents a very cost-effective option in the prevention and management of chronic diseases in young people.

This chapter addresses the importance of physical activity for children's growth and development with implications for overweight and obesity. Recognition of the importance of physical activity to the health and well-being of all young people is of paramount importance to all parents, teachers, health professionals and carers of young children.

Physical activity and obesity prevention in youngsters

Physical activity is widely recognised as essential for the normal growth and development of children and youth. Participation in regular physical activity also contributes to a lower risk of obesity, coronary heart disease, hypertension, type 2 diabetes, colon cancer, osteoarthritis, and osteoporosis in adulthood. Not surprisingly, physical activity has long been described as public health's 'best buy' (van Mechelen, 1997) particularly as the persistence of childhood overweight into adulthood is associated with more severe obesity among adults.

The dramatic increases in the prevalence of childhood overweight and obesity, plus the potential effect on morbidity and mortality at all stages in the lifespan, highlight the need for a better understanding of the role of physical activity in weight management. A useful starting point is to be aware of 'critical periods' during the growing years, times when the risk of onset, complications or persistence of overweight and obesity is increased (Dietz, 2004). Critical periods during the formative years are infancy, early childhood and adolescence, times of rapid growth and development and transition.

Critical periods of growth and development may also be consistent with times when additional emphasis should be placed on physical activity (Hills, 1995). This may be the case, for example, in the transition from childhood to adolescence, when activity levels may decline in many youngsters. Additional times of vulnerability may include the early childhood years, the beginning of school, and the transition from elementary school to high school (Sallis, 2000), and between school and the workforce or higher education (Gordon-Larsen, 2004). In short, insufficient levels of physical activity at any stage during the growing years are a major contributing factor to overweight and obesity.

In relation to the current obesity epidemic, Olshansky *et al.* (2005) have suggested that 'the youth of today may, on average, live less healthy and possibly even shorter lives than their parents.'

In addition, an understanding of the more common contributing factors to excess weight gain and poor body composition during childhood and adolescence is central to effective prevention and management of overweight and obesity. The ideal foundation would be for all children to be provided with the chance to develop the motor skills necessary for meaningful involvement in physical activity.

Consistent with the encouragement to increase physical activity levels in young people should be the development of innovative approaches to reduce inactive behaviours (Parízková and Hills, 2005). A coordinated approach is required by parents, teachers, and health professionals to influence the knowledge, attitudes and behaviours of youngsters. The establishment of desirable lifestyle behaviours early in life is an important goal as there is a strong likelihood that the nature of an individual's exposure to nutrition and physical activity, combined with genetic predisposition to increased weight gain, may influence changes in growth and unhealthy development of weight and its complications (Yanovski and Yanovski, 2003).

At the population level, physical activity promotion strategies need to emphasise community capacity and sustainability. In addition, to maximise the benefits from physical activity and exercise in the context of body composition and weight management, more of an emphasis is needed on matching activity promotion strategies for the population with optimal exercise prescription for the individual.

The ideal scenario would be to prevent the development of overweight and obesity in young people.

Physical activity during the growing years

Despite the well-documented benefits of physical activity to health, fitness and normal growth and development of young people, an increasing proportion of the childhood population is overweight or obese. It is apparent that lip-service is being paid to the area, and in particular, physical activity and body composition. This lack of awareness and inaction appears to be most pronounced in relation to children of pre-school age.

Of particular concern is that many young children do not participate in appropriate levels of physical activity. Low levels of habitual physical activity and energy expenditure plus poor eating behaviours in young children are major determinants of obesity. The persistence of these conditions in young people helps to perpetuate a 'vicious cycle' of limited physical activity experiences, sedentary behaviours and poor eating habits.

It is never too early to foster appropriate activity opportunities and eating behaviours. For example, if the goal is to adopt quality lifestyle practices in all young people from birth, sound knowledge and understanding of expectant mothers in the area is a basic requirement. A coordinated approach to the prevention and management of overweight and obesity is needed from all adults who influence the knowledge, attitudes and behaviours of young people. This group includes parents, health professionals, caregivers and teachers.

As very young children are dependent on responsible adults for guidance, adults must be role models for acceptable behaviour and also recognise the individual needs of children. Further, adults need to appreciate the importance of safe and enjoyable physical activity so that activity is a central platform in the growth and development of all children.

The importance of physical activity to normal growth and development, including the health and well-being of children and youth, is widely acknowledged (AIHW, 2003; Borms, 1986; Caine and Maffulli, 2005; Chakravarthy and Booth, 2004). In particular, regular physical activity has been associated with the maintenance of optimal metabolic function (Chakravarthy and Booth, 2004; Cordain *et al.*, 1998; Eaton, Conner and Shostak, 1988) and the prevention of chronic disease (Booth *et al.*, 2002). Related benefits of regular weight-bearing activity include its contribution to the maintenance of skeletal health and desirable body composition by controlling weight and minimising body fat (USDHHS, 1996). Further, regular physical activity participation plays a key role in social and mental development (Hill, 2005). Most importantly, activity has also been associated with psycho-social benefits including a reduction in the symptoms of depression, stress, anxiety (Dunn, Trivedi and O'Neal, 2001), and improvements in self-confidence and self-esteem.

During the growing years, adjustments in health and motor-related components of fitness are influenced by growth and maturation. Therefore, it is difficult to

separate the impact of regular participation in physical activity during the formative years from the adjustments in growth and development (Hills, 1995).

Both nutrition and physical activity influence the growth and development
of growing children (Meredith and Dwyer, 1991). However, growth and maturation will continue despite limited physical activity (Malina, 2000), whereas sound
nutrition (ideally combined with physical activity) is essential to maximise growth
and development. Consequently, when nutrition and physical activity is optimal,
growth and development of youngsters is more likely to match their genetic potential. Unfortunately, in today's society the opportunities for many youngsters to
be physically active are often limited, commonly owing to environmental factors
(Dollman and Norton, 2005).

A cost-effective way to prevent or minimise the risk of obesity and related
chronic diseases would be to combine sound nutritional practices with adequate
levels of physical activity (Meredith and Dwyer, 1991). To be successful, such an
approach needs to be employed from birth and engage all sectors of society, in
particular health professionals, teachers and parents. An integral component is for
responsible adults to have an appreciation of the normal individual variability in
physical growth in relation to body size, shape and composition (Rogol, Clark and
Roemmich, 2000). Young children are dependent on responsible adults for guidance regarding acceptable behaviour. Adults need to be aware of the importance
of enjoyment in physical activity and the environmental factors that have a potent
influence on children's physical activity (Franks *et al.*, 2005; Moore *et al.*, 1995).
In short, parents' attitudes, the encouragement of family-based activity, and the
provision of opportunities to facilitate activity should be considered (Mullan, Dan
ielzi and Pust, 2005).

Many authors have suggested that spontaneous physical activity has been 'engineered' out of the modern lifestyle, particularly in the developed world (Chakravarthy and Booth, 2004), commonly in combination with poor nutrition. Recent
reports of trends in developing countries identify the combination of underweight
children and overweight adults, often in the same family (Caballero, 2004).

There are still gaps in our knowledge and understanding of the relationship
between regular physical activity during the growing years and impact on adult
health. Despite this, most would support the contention that adult health benefits,
particularly those related to body composition, are associated with the commence-
ment of habitual physical activity from a young age (Twisk, 2001). In contrast,
the early incorporation of physical inactivity into daily life contributes to chronic
health problems (Booth *et al.*, 2002; Chakravarthy and Booth, 2004; Paffenbarger
et al., 1986). Interestingly, the suggestion of a threshold of physical activity has
recently been hypothesised by Chakravarthy and Booth (2004). Activity levels
below such a threshold may imply a 'physical activity deficiency' (Chakravarthy
and Booth, 2003).

Regular physical activity and normal motor development

The early years of life should be the time of motor learning foundation for all children and the subsequent development of progressively more complex skills. During the childhood years, individuals who are more physically active have the opportunity to further refine their motor skills (Graf *et al.*, 2004). Through active play, young children develop the fundamental movement patterns of crawling, standing, walking, running and jumping. However, restrictions in physical activity opportunities may jeopardise skill development and compromise body composition as a result of lower levels of energy expenditure (Booth *et al.*, 2005). In short, movement provides the ideal opportunity for youngsters to explore the environment and their physical capabilities, and most children relish the opportunity to participate in progressively more vigorous and physically challenging activities.

Differences in the individual patterns of growth and development are largely responsible for the variability in timing of motor milestones. This variability may also contribute to specific characteristics such as the rewards of physical activity, including enhanced self-esteem, self-confidence and competence. Activity experiences also provide children with sensory information through visual, tactile and auditory mechanisms, as well as from vestibular and kinaesthetic receptors. Gallahue (1982) has suggested that young children engage in movement activities that may be categorised as tasks of 'learning to move' and 'learning through movement'. Both play important roles in the overall growth and development of children.

The early establishment of appropriate lifestyle practices in young children is more important than the reinforcement of sedentary behaviours (Epstein *et al.*, 1999); however, environmental factors often favour inactive lifestyles (Franklin, 2001). Positive activity opportunities are more likely to facilitate fun and enjoyment and subsequent spontaneity and pleasure in movement for young people (Barrett, 2001). Hills (1995) contends that success in the activity setting may be one of the defining features in the establishment of longer-term habitual physical activity and a healthy body composition. Physical competency may also be a strong factor in the likelihood of participation in physical activity in later years (Gately *et al.*, 2000; Reynolds *et al.*, 1990; Walker *et al.*, 2003).

Early childhood is also a prime time for the establishment of social behaviours. However, during this period, children are dependent on responsible adults, including for their opportunities to participate in physical activity. In relation to participation in activity and physical performance, most children make the transition from being self-centred to seeking assistance and approval from significant others, including their parents. Children's participation in more vigorous social play behaviours such as wrestling, kicking and tumbling are very much influenced by adult involvement, or lack of it. Commonly, the earliest experiences of these types of activities are facilitated by a parent, more often the father. Participation in more vigorous types of play generally peaks at approximately 8–10 years of age. The quality of the early activity experiences of young children influences the rewards of activity participation including improvements in self-esteem and self-confidence, plus feelings of mastery and competence. Experiencing success and enjoyment in activity is consistent with the likelihood of young people continuing to seek to be active.

Physical activity and public health challenges

Despite the increasing recognition of the benefits of physical activity, too many children and adults, particularly in developed countries, are inactive (AIHW, 2004). Key environmental drivers for inactivity in children include technologies and parental concerns regarding safety. The protectiveness of parents means that restrictions are often placed on where children play and also the likelihood of walking or cycling to and from school. In Australia for example, active transport levels of children are very low (Harten and Olds, 2004) and playing computer games and watching television and DVDs/videos are very popular among children (ABS, 2001).

The highest public health priority in the context of overweight and obesity should be to promote the importance of physical activity in children and match this with increased opportunities to be active. There is an urgent need for a well-resourced, comprehensive, population-based set of strategies to increase physical activity to address the obesity problem. Action areas should include multi-strategy, multi-setting intervention programmes; community-wide communications programmes; national coordination of prevention effort and capacity building; and the appropriate and sustained training of health professionals.

By necessity, the public health physical activity messages to date have commonly been simplistic and generic. Messages have related to physical activity and health and largely focused on the adult population. Similarly, less attention has been paid to the prevention of weight gain or weight regain, to weight loss and, particularly, to the implications for children and adolescents (Saris *et al.*, 2003).

For adults, the consistent public health message related to physical activity and health has been to accumulate 30 minutes or more of moderate-intensity physical activity on most, preferably all, days of the week. For children and youth the recommendation has been to participate in at least 60 minutes of activity per day. An ongoing challenge for the field is to maximise the population's exposure to and understanding of such messages, including the interpretation of ambiguous terms such as 'moderate-intensity'. Just as important is the recognition that added benefits can be gained by individuals, groups and the wider population if the generic recommendations are complemented by additional guidance regarding intensity, duration and frequency of physical activity and exercise.

In addition, a relatively conservative approach has commonly been employed in recommending the volume of exercise necessary for the maintenance of desirable body composition or, where necessary, weight loss. In overweight and obese children, the goal should be to increase physical activity and exercise, not necessarily to focus on weight loss. It is important to acknowledge that the current public health messages regarding physical activity and the importance of increasing incidental physical activity are a good starting point for the improvement of health status, particularly in individuals who are inactive. However, to gain maximum benefits, a progressive increase in the individualised exercise dose is needed to optimise health and weight maintenance, or weight loss if needed. This applies to individuals of all ages.

Physical activity recommendations for children: what is the evidence?

Despite the well-established relationship between physical activity and health benefits (Bauman, 2004), and the increasing prevalence of childhood obesity, there has been little attention paid to evidence-based physical activity recommendations for young people in the recent past (Goran, Reynolds and Lindquist, 1999; van Mechelen *et al.*, 2000; Wareham *et al.*, 2005).

However, a recent review by Strong *et al.* (2005) has both summarised data on physical activity and health in children and also recommended a minimum of 60 min/day of moderate to vigorous activity. This recommendation is consistent with the advice of other groups (Cavill, Biddle and Sallis, 2001; CDC, 1997; Department of Health, 2004; Sallis and Patrick, 1994). As for adult activity recommendations, there has been considerable confusion regarding guidelines for cardiorespiratory health and body composition (prevention or treatment of weight gain) benefits (Blair, LaMonte and Nichaman, 2004; Saris *et al.*, 2003). Recommendations for children should not necessarily focus on weight management or other specific health benefits but rather encourage a significant increase in physical activity, particularly active play in very young children (Burdette and Whitaker, 2005).

All children and adolescents should be physically active daily. Physical activity opportunities for young people may be part of play, school physical education, sport, games, active transport (for example walking and cycling to school), recreation, and planned exercise. Activity may be undertaken in the context of the family, school, and wider community setting.

Consistent with the message that all children and youth should engage in physical activity of at least moderate intensity for 60 minutes or more each day should be the avoidance of extended periods of inactivity. This includes sedentary behaviours such as watching television, DVDs and videos, playing computer games or surfing the internet. As for inactive adults, inactive youngsters should commence activity by participating in shorter periods of moderate-intensity activity and progressively build to the goal of 60 minutes per day.

Despite the lack of evidence for specific long-term benefits associated with physical activity participation in childhood and youth, there are compelling reasons for supporting an activity recommendation that is higher than the public health recommendation for adults. The more obvious reasons relate to the extent of the obesity epidemic in young people, and the increasing evidence that low levels of physical activity and increased engagement in sedentary pursuits are major contributing factors to increased body fatness over time.

Summary

Despite the lack of empirical evidence to support definitive physical activity guidelines for children and adolescents, a physically active lifestyle is consistent with positive health and the prevention of disease (Chakravarthy and Booth, 2004), and a sedentary lifestyle is associated with chronic disease and ill health (Twisk, 2001; Westerterp, 1999). Physical activity levels in young people are influenced by a range of factors, in particular the environment. Greater attention needs to be paid to preventing more children becoming overweight and obese, including through environmental and policy changes in children and adolescents (Robinson and Sirard, 2005; Wilkin and Voss, 2004).

References

ABS (Australian Bureau of Statistics) (2001) *Children's Participation in Cultural and Leisure Activities, Australia*, cat. no. 4901.0, Canberra: ABS.

AIHW (Australian Institute of Health and Welfare) (2003) *Australia's Young People*, Canberra: AIHW.

AIHW (Australian Institute of Health and Welfare) (2004) *A Rising Epidemic: Overweight and Obesity in Australian Children and Adolescents*, Risk Factors Data Briefing 2, Canberra: AIHW.

Barrett, B.J. (2001) 'Play now, play later. Lifetime fitness implications', *Journal of Physical Education, Recreation and Dance*, 72(8): 35–9.

Bauman, A.E. (2004) 'Updating the evidence that physical activity is good for health: an epidemiological review 2000–2003', *Journal of Science and Medicine in Sports*, 1: 6–19.

Blair, S.N., LaMonte, M.J. and Nichaman, M.Z. (2004) 'The evolution of physical activity recommendations: how much is enough?', *American Journal of Clinical Nutrition*, 79: 913–20S.

Booth, F.W., Chakravarthy, M.V., Gordon, S.E. and Spangenburg, E.E. (2002) 'Waging war on physical inactivity: using modern molecular ammunition against an ancient enemy', *Journal of Applied Physiology*, 93: 3–30.

Booth, K.M., Pinkston, M.M. and Poston, W.S. (2005) 'Obesity and the built environment', *Journal of the American Dietetic Association*, 105(5 Suppl 1): S110–17.

Borms, J. (1986) 'Children and exercise: an overview', *Journal of Sports Sciences*, 4: 3–20.

Burdette, H.L. and Whitaker, R.C. (2005) 'Resurrecting free play in young children: looking beyond fitness and fatness attention, affiliation and affect', *Archives of Pediatric and Adolescent Medicine*, 159(1): 46–50.

Caballero, B. (2004) 'A nutrition paradox – undernutrition and obesity in developing countries', *New England Journal of Medicine*, 352(15): 1514–16.

Caine, D. and Maffulli, N. (2005) 'Epidemiology of children's individual sports injuries', in D.J. Caine, N. Maffulli (eds) *Epidemiology of Pediatric Sports Injuries. Individual Sports*, Basel: Medicine and Sport Science, Karger, vol. 48, pp. 1–7.

Cavill, N., Biddle, S. and Sallis, J.F. (2001) 'Health-enhancing physical activity for young people: statement of the United Kingdom Expert Consensus Conference', *Pediatric Exercise Science*, 13: 12–25.

CDC (Centers for Disease Control and Prevention) (1997) 'Guidelines for school and community programmes to promote lifelong physical activity among young people', *Morbidity and Mortality Weekly Report*, 46: 1–36.

Chakravarthy, M.V. and Booth, F.W. (2003) *Exercise*, Philadelphia, PA: Elsevier.

Chakravarthy, M.V. and Booth, F.W. (2004) 'Eating, exercise, and "thrifty" genotypes: connecting the dots toward an evolutionary understanding of modern chronic diseases', *Journal of Applied Physiology*, 96: 3–10.

Cordain, L., Gotshall, R.W., Eaton, S.B. and Eaton, S.B. III (1998) 'Physical activity, energy expenditure and fitness: an evolutionary perspective', *International Journal of Sports Medicine*, 19: 328–35.

Department of Health (2004) *Physical Activity, Health Improvement and Prevention. At Least Five a Week*, London: Department of Health, UK.

Dietz, W.H. (2004) 'Overweight in childhood and adolescence', *New England Journal of Medicine*, 18(4): 312–15.

Dollman, J. and Norton, K. (2005) 'Evidence for secular trends in children's physical activity behaviour', *British Journal of Sports Medicine*, 39: 892–7.

Dunn, A.L., Trivedi, M.H. and O'Neal, H.A. (2001) 'Physical activity dose-response effects on outcomes of depression and anxiety', *Medicine and Science in Sports and Exercise*, 33(6 Suppl): S587–97; discussion 609–10.

Eaton, S.B., Conner, M. and Shostak, M. (1988) 'Stone agers in the fast lane: chronic degenerative diseases in evolutionary perspective', *American Journal of Medicine*, 84: 739–49.

Epstein, L.H., Paluch, R.A., Gordy, C.C. and Dorn, J. (1999) 'Reinforcing value of physical activity as a determinant of child activity level', *Health Psychology*, 18: 599–603.

Franklin, B.A. (2001) 'The downside of our technological revolution? An obesity-conducive environment', *American Journal of Cardiology*, 87(9): 1093–5.

Franks, P.W., Ravussin, E., Hanso, R.L., Harper, I.T., Allison, D.B., Knowler, W.C., Tatarani, P.A. and Salbe, A.D. (2005) 'Habitual physical activity in children: the role of genes and environment', *American Journal of Clinical Nutrition*, 82: 901–8.

Gallahue, D.L. (1982) *Understanding Motor Development in Children*, New York: John Wiley and Sons.

Gately, P.J., Cooke, C.B., Butterly, R.J., Mackreth, P. and Carroll, S. (2000) 'The effects of a children's summer camp programme on weight loss, with a 10 month follow-up', *International Journal of Obesity and Related Metabolic Disorders*, 24(11): 1445–52.

Goran, M.I., Reynolds, K.D. and Lindquist, C.H. (1999) 'Role of physical activity in the prevention of obesity in children', *International Journal of Obesity and Related Metabolic Disorders*, 23(3): S18–33.

Gordon-Larsen, P., Adair, L.S., Nelson, M.C. and Popkin, B.M. (2004) 'Five year obesity incidence in the transition period between adolescence and adulthood: the National Longitudinal Study of Adolescent Health', *American Journal of Clinical Nutrition*, 80: 569–75.

Graf, C., Koch, B., Kretschmann-Kandel, E., Falkowski, G., Christ, H., Coburger, S., Lehmacher, W., Bjarnason-Wehrens, B., Platen, P., Tokarski, W., Predel, H.G., Dordel, S. (2004) 'Correlation between BMI, leisure habits and motor abilities in childhood', *International Journal of Obesity*, 28: 22–6.

Harten, N. and Olds, T. (2004) 'Patterns of active transport in 11–12 year old Australian children', *Australian and New Zealand Journal of Public Health*, 28(2): 167–72.

Hill, A. (2005) 'Social and self-perception of obese children and adolescents', in N. Caero, N.G. Norgan, G.T.H. Ellison (eds) *Childhood Obesity*, London: Taylor & Francis, pp. 39–49.

Hills, A.P. (1995) 'Physical activity and movement in children: its consequences for growth and development', *Asia Pacific Journal of Clinical Nutrition*, 4: 43–5.

Malina, R.M. (2000) 'Growth and maturation: do regular physical activity and training for sport have a significant influence?', in N. Armstrong, W. van Mechelen (eds) *Paediatric Exercise Science and Medicine*, Oxford: Oxford University Press, pp. 95–106.

van Mechelen, W. (1997) 'A physically active lifestyle – public health's best buy', *British Journal of Sports Medicine*, 31(4): 264–5.

van Mechelen, W., Twisk, J.W.R., Post, G.B., Snel, J. and Kemper, H.C.G. (2000) 'Physical activity of young people: the Amsterdam Longitudinal Growth and Health Study', *Medicine and Science in Sports and Exercise*, 32(9): 1610–16.

Meredith, C.N. and Dwyer, J.T. (1991) 'Nutrition and exercise: effects on adolescent health', *Annual Reviews of Public Health*, 12: 309–33.

Moore, L.L., Nguyen, U.S.D.T., Rothman, K.J. and Ellison, R.C. (1995) 'Preschool physical activity level and change in body fatness in young children. The Framingham Children's Study', *American Journal of Epidemiology*, 142(9): 982–8.

Muller, M.J., Danielzi, S. and Pust, S. (2005) 'School- and family-based interventions to prevent overweight children', *Proceedings of the Nutrition Society*, 64: 249–54.

Olshansky, S.J., Passaro, D.J., Hershow, R.C., Layden, J., Carnes, B.A., Brody, J., Hayflick, L., Butler, R.N., Allison, D.B. and Ludwig, D.S. (2005) 'A potential decline in life expectancy in the United States in the 21st century', *New England Journal of Medicine*, 352(11): 1138–45.

Paffenbarger, R.S., Hyde, R.T., Wing, A.L. and Hsieh, C.C. (1986) 'Physical activity, all-cause mortality and longevity of college alumni', *New England Journal of Medicine*, 314: 605–13.

Parízková, J. and Hills, A.P. (2005) *Childhood Obesity: Prevention and Management*, 2nd edition, Boca Raton, FL: CRC Press.

Reilly, J.J. and McDowell, Z.C. (2003) 'Physical activity interventions in the prevention and treatment of paediatric obesity: systematic review and critical appraisal', *Proceedings of the Nutrition Society*, 62: 611–19.

Reynolds, K., Killen, J.D., Beyson, S.W., Maron, D.J., Taylor, C.D., Maccoby, N. and Farquar, J.W. (1990) 'Psychosocial predictors of physical activity in adolescents', *Preventive Medicine*, 19: 541–51.

Robinson, T.N. and Sirard, J.R. (2005) 'Preventing childhood obesity. A solution-orientated research paradigm', *American Journal of Preventive Medicine*, 28: 194–201.

Rogol, A.D., Clark, P.A. and Roemmich, J.N. (2000) 'Growth and pubertal development in children and adolescents: effects of diet and physical activity', *American Journal of Clinical Nutrition*, 72(Suppl): S521–S528.

Sallis, J.F. and Patrick, K. (1994) 'Physical activity guidelines for adolescents: consensus statement', *Pediatric Exercise Science*, 6: 302–14.

Sallis, J.F. (2000) 'A review of correlates of physical activity of children and adolescents', *Medicine and Science in Sports and Exercise*, 32: 963–75.

Saris, W.H., Blair, S.N., van Baak, M.A., Eaton, S.B., Davies, P.S.W., Di Pietro, L., Fogelholm, M., Rissanen, A., Schoeller, D., Swinburn, B., Tremblay, A., Westerterp, K.R. and Wyatt, H. (2003) 'How much physical activity is enough to prevent unhealthy weight gain? Outcome of the IASO 1st Stock Conference and consensus statement', *Obesity Reviews*, 4(2): 101–14.

Strong, W.B., Malina, R.M., Blimkie, C.J.R., Daniels, S.R., Dishman, R.K., Gutin, B., Hergenroeder, A.C., Must, A., Nixon, P.A., Pivarnik, J.M., Rowland, T., Trost, S. and Trudeau, F. (2005) 'Evidence based physical activity for school-age youth', *Journal of Pediatrics*, 146: 732–7.

Twisk, J.W.R. (2001) 'Physical activity guidelines for children and adolescents. A critical review', *Sports Medicine*, 31(8): 617–27.

USDHHS (United States Department of Health and Human Services) (1996) *Physical Activity and Health: A Report of the Surgeon General.* Atlanta, GA: Centers for Disease Control and Prevention.

Walker, L.L., Gately, P.J., Bewick, B.M. and Hill, A.J. (2003) 'Children's weight-loss camps: psychological benefit or jeopardy', *International Journal of Obesity and Related Metabolic Disorders*, 27(6): 748–54.

Wareham, N.J., Esther, M.F., van Sluijs, E.M.F. and Ekelund, U. (2005) 'Physical activity and obesity prevention: a review of the current evidence', *Proceedings of the Nutrition Society*, 64: 229–47.

Westerterp, K.R. (1999) 'Assessment of physical activity level in relation to obesity: current evidence and research issues', *Medicine and Science in Sports and Exercise*, 31: S522–5.

Wilkin, T. and Voss, L.D. (2004) 'Physical activity in young children', *Lancet*, 363(9415): 1162–3.

Yanovski, J.A. and Yanovski, S.Z. (2003) 'Treatment of pediatric and adolescent obesity', *Journal of the American Medical Association*, 289(14): 1851–3.

6 The role of perceived competence in the motivation of obese children to be physically active

L.M. Lyell, S.C. Wearing and A.P. Hills

Introduction

Targeted promotion of physical activity in youth has been advocated as an ideal method to combat the worldwide rise in childhood obesity and is thought to maximize the continuation of active behaviours through adolescence and into adulthood. Although the heath benefits of physical activity have been widely touted, recognition of the benefits of physical activity for the overweight and obese is not sufficient. The major challenge remains to motivate individuals to participate in physical activity and to provide the necessary support to maximize enjoyment and adherence. This chapter provides an overview of the role of perceived competence and self-concept in the motivation of obese children to participate in physical activity. It also provides recommendations regarding the design and delivery of programmes that promote physical activity by enhancing the perceived competence of the obese child.

Background

The increasing prevalence of childhood obesity and the corresponding reduction in physical activity in young people has led to a heightened interest in strategies designed to prevent and manage the condition (Elliott, Copperman and Jacobson, 2004; Flodmark *et al.*, 2004). Research suggests that appropriate eating and exercise behaviours should be integral to any management strategy (Rowland, 2004; Steinbeck, 2001; Stunkard, 1996). The benefits of physical activity and exercise for children and youth have been well documented and parallel those reported for adults. Benefits include a decreased risk of cardiovascular disease, improved physical capabilities and an increased sense of well-being (Hills, 1998; Taylor and Sallis, 1997). The opportunity and encouragement for all children to be physically active from a young age may help to maximize the continuation of active behaviours through adolescence and into adulthood (Baranowski *et al.*, 2000). This practice would be beneficial at both the individual and population levels. However, recognition of the benefits of physical activity for the overweight and obese is not sufficient. The major challenge remains to motivate individuals to participate in physical activity and to provide the necessary support to maximize enjoyment and adherence. Evidence suggests that overprescribing exercise intensity results in a reduction in self-reported pleasure in overweight individuals (Ekkekakis and Lind, 2006) and that the perceived tolerance and pleasure (i.e. affective response) of physical activity influence compliance (Ekkekakis, Hall and Petrizzello, 2005). Therefore, the affective (i.e. pleasure) response associated with exercise has important implications for adoption and adherence. If one accepts the premise that physical activity is central to the weight management process in overweight and obese children (Baranowski *et al.*, 2000), then how important is the relationship between competence and motivation to exercise participation in this population?

In the activity setting, the obese child is commonly disadvantaged compared with normal-weight peers. The obese individual is disadvantaged by physical (i.e. body weight) and cardiovascular constraints, particularly during weight-bearing tasks. This may be further complicated by psychosocial constraints (Hills, 1994; Myers and Rosen, 1999; Neumark-Sztainer, Story and Faibisch, 1998; Parízková *et al.*, 1994.). For example, it is not uncommon for the overweight child to be teased and berated by others and for this to contribute to a reduction in self-esteem, a dislike of physical activity and a subsequent lack of desire to exercise (Mulvihill, Rivers and Aggleton, 2000). Data also suggest that obese and overweight girls have lower physical appearance and athletic competence self-esteem compared with lean girls (Phillips and Hill, 1998). Figure 6.1 outlines the psychological and physical barriers experienced by obese children. Collectively, these barriers contribute to a lowering of the tolerance of physical activity in obese children. It is important to be aware of these barriers when promoting physical activity in children. (Also see the discussion in Chapter 7.) Overcoming these complications in the obese

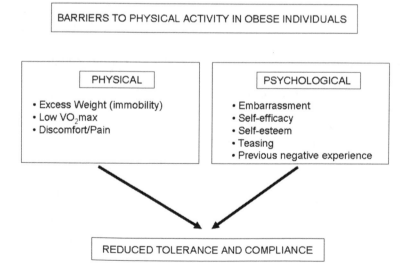

Figure 6.1 A schematic diagram outlining the potential barriers associated with physical activity in obese individuals.

pediatric population should be a major goal for educators, health professionals, parents and others working in the area of childhood obesity (Neumark-Sztainer, Story and Faibisch, 1998).

The primary aim of this chapter is to provide an amalgamation of the contemporary information in the area of perceived competence and self-concept, and to report on the role of these constructs in the motivation of obese children to participate in physical activity. A further aim is to explore how the design and delivery of physical activity programmes and exercise experiences can be improved to enhance the perceived competence of the obese child. Because of the paucity of work in this area with the obese, research findings with normal-weight children have been considered and the implications for the obese population assessed.

Definitions and models

The concept of perceived competence or perceived ability has been a central thesis in numerous motivational theories, with various researchers proposing models to explain behaviour in an achievement context. Harter's (1981) Competence Motivation Theory has gained widespread acceptance and, in particular, the Self Perception Profile for Children has been widely used in contemporary research. However, other models, such as the Achievement Goal Theory proposed by Nicholls and Miller (1984) and the Expectancy–Value Theory proposed by Eccles *et al.* (1983) have also considered perceptions of competence to be integral to motivation in the sport and exercise setting. These models and the role that perceived competence plays in each will be briefly reviewed in the context of physical activity.

Competence motivation theory

Harter's Competence Motivation Theory posits that 'individuals will be motivated to engage in tasks when they perceive themselves to be competent and conversely withdraw from activities when they perceive that they lack competence' (Solmon *et al.*, 2003: 261). Harter initially proposed that children as young as eight years of age make meaningful differentiations among cognitive, social and physical competencies and also have defined opinions about their general self-worth. However, Harter (1990) later revised this theory and identified scholastic competence, athletic competence, peer acceptance, physical appearance and behavioural conduct as domains in which children make competence judgments. These judgments are used to form their overall self-concept, which in turn mediates their affective, motivational and behavioural states (see Figure 6.2). Harter contends that important psychological correlates impact on domain-specific perceived competence: namely the child's locus of control and motivational orientation (Harter and Connell, 1984). Thus, a child who is intrinsically motivated in a particular task is also likely to perceive themselves as competent in that task and in control of success or failure.

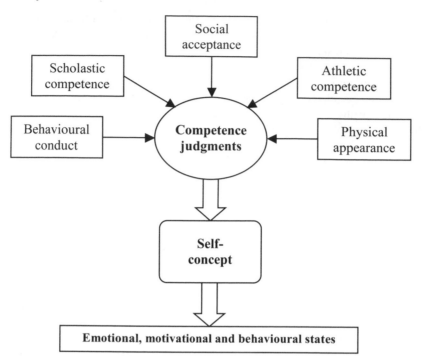

Figure 6.2   Illustration of the Competence Motivation Theory. Discrepancies between perceptions of competence in the domains of *physical appearance, social acceptance, behavioural conduct* and *scholastic* and *athletic competence* and the importance placed on success in these domains are systematically correlated with global self-esteem. Self-esteem, in turn, mediates affective motivational and behavioural states.

Achievement goal theory

Nicholls and Miller's (1984) Achievement Goal Theory suggests that perceived competence is the goal of behaviour and a person's concept of their ability and definitions of success will influence the activities in which they choose to engage. Integral to this theory are the notions of goal orientations and conception of ability. Two orthogonal goal orientations, termed 'task' and 'ego', relate to the individual's definition of success. A person who possesses a task orientation defines success in terms of mastery of the task, whereas an ego-oriented person defines success in terms of demonstrating superior ability relative to others. In turn, conception of ability reflects an individual's differentiation of the concept of effort from ability. A person with a differentiated concept of ability views ability as capacity unaffected by effort, whereas a person with an undifferentiated concept of ability believes effort equals ability and therefore the more effort expended in completing a task the higher the perceived ability (Nicholls, 1989). Williams and Gill (1995) tested the relationship between goal orientations, perceived competence, intrinsic interest and effort and found that task orientation, perceived competence and intrinsic interest accounted for 41 per cent of the variance in effort. Several studies have confirmed this positive relationship between task orientation, higher levels of perceived competence and participation variables (Fox *et al.*, 1994; Roberts, Kleiber and Duda, 1981; Stephens, 1998).

Goal orientations are influenced by two motivational climates, most commonly described as mastery- or performance-oriented climates that emphasize the task and ego goals, respectively. A number of studies (Ebbeck and Weiss, 1998; Theeboom, De Knop and Weiss, 1995; Treasure, 1997; Williams and Gill, 1995; Xiang and Lee, 1998) have investigated the interaction between motivational climate, conceptions of physical ability and perceived ability and confirmed that individuals who perceive a high mastery climate in an activity setting hold high perceptions of ability and believe that effort is directly related to success in that setting.

The expectancy–value model

The expectancy–value model proposed by Eccles *et al.* (1983) argues that a combination of the individual's expectancy of success and the value attached to a particular task is an important predictor of an individual's choice to engage in an activity. The model also includes such factors as usefulness, enjoyment, importance and gender-role schemata, and theorizes that, when children devalue an activity and have low competence beliefs about it, they will be less likely to engage in it. Further, Shapiro and Ulrich (2002) studied the relationship between perceived task value and perceived competence in children and found significant relationships between each of the components of task value and perceived competence. Specifically, enjoyment, importance and usefulness were all significantly correlated with perceived competence.

Perceived competence is also central to intrinsic motivation in the Self Determination Theory (Deci and Ryan, 1985), with perceived locus of causality and perceived competence identified as responsible for changes in intrinsic motivation. This theory is similar to Attribution Theory, which posits that after experiencing success or failure individuals search for explanations for the outcome, with such attribution interpretations partly determining subsequent affective reactions, which in turn impact on motivational behaviour (Weiner, 1986). Sinnott and Biddle (1998) were able to support this theory, albeit in a small sample of children who received attribution retraining after failure at an achievement task. Following attribution retraining and a repeat of the task, measures of perceived success and intrinsic motivation were significantly higher for all children in the experimental group and all children made internal and controllable attributions for the outcome of their attempts.

Therefore, perceived competence has been identified as a central construct in most theories of motivation. In the context of the increasing prevalence of childhood obesity, it is important to establish how perceived competence and related constructs operate in this population and further, to determine how to support children to become intrinsically motivated and adopt physical activity as a lifelong habit.

Perceived competence and physical activity in the obese child

Relatively few studies have specifically examined the impact of weight on perceived physical competence in children. Despite the lack of conclusive evidence of the relationship between weight or adiposity and perceptions of competence, there appears to be sufficient evidence to encourage further research. A recent study of actual and perceived competence in normal-weight and overweight children found significantly lower perceived physical competence and significantly lower actual total competence and locomotion competence in the overweight (Southall, Okely and Steele, 2004). Similarly, Phillips and Hill (1998), using Harter's Self Perception Profile for Children, found that weight had a significant impact on overall perceived competence with the most apparent effects being on athletic competence and physical appearance. These findings are consistent with the study by Braet, Mervielde and Vandereycken (1997), who found that clinical and non-clinical obese individuals were significantly lower on physical and self-worth scales than the control group. The degree of overweight impacted on perceived competence with both physical competence and self-worth being negatively correlated with degree of overweight.

Given the limited research on perceived competence in the obese population, two examples of studies with participants who face similar difficulties to the obese will be used to further illustrate the role of this construct. Rose, Larkin and Berger (1997) investigated perceived competence in a group of poorly coordinated children using a well-coordinated group as controls. The poorly coordinated group had significantly lower perceptions of physical competence and social acceptance than those who were well-coordinated. Similar results were reported by Causgrove Dunn (2000) in an examination of goal orientations, perceptions of the motivational climate and perceived competence in a group of children with movement difficulties. The dispositional tendency to adopt task-involved goals was positively related to the perception of a mastery motivational climate, which in turn was positively related to perceived competence.

It appears that overweight or obesity is related to lower perceived competence; the actual competence of the obese child is also likely to be reduced. It has been suggested that obesity can result from, and be the cause of, decreased physical activity in children (Brownell, 1995; Davies, Gregory and White, 1995). Davies, Gregory and White (1995) reported that decreased physical activity was significantly correlated to percentage body fat in non-obese pre-school children; a finding supported by later research that BMI is a significant negative predictor of physical activity (Craig, Goldberg and Dietz, 1996). Epstein *et al.* (1996) examined determinants of physical activity in obese children and found fitness measured by a sub-maximal VO_2 test accounted for 23 per cent of the variance in self-reported activity, which provides further support for this suggestion. Additional research is warranted to establish to what extent actual physical competence predicts activity in obese children. In addition to lower perceived competence, obese children suffer from other psychosocial effects, which can lead to decreased self-esteem and psychopathology (Kaplan and Wadden, 1986; Korsch, 1986; Neumark-Sztainer, Story and Faibisch, 1998; Phillips and Hill, 1998), the results of which may influence physical activity. For example, Neumark-Sztainer, Story and Faibisch (1998) found that overweight adolescent girls were most frequently stigmatized through direct and intentional stigmatizing behaviour. Research by Pierce and Wardell (1997) revealed that, in addition to stigmatization, obese children had lower global and appearance self-esteem than non-obese children. Conversely, Kaplan and Wadden (1986) measured global self-esteem in a sample of black children and adolescents and found that the overweight and obese subjects did not differ from normal-weight subjects on global self-esteem, but found that leanness was associated with enhanced self-worth. Interestingly, parental concern about weight status can affect self-esteem and perceived physical ability in the negative direction (Davison and Birch, 2001). Davison and Birch (2001) discovered that, although girls with higher weight status had lower body esteem, there was no relationship between their weight status and perceived physical ability. However, concern about weight status on the part of the mother (independent of weight status) was associated with lower perceived physical ability. This research confirms the multiple variables that combine to determine a child's self-esteem and perceived competence, and highlights the impact of the obese child's social environment on their self-worth.

In summary, despite the lack of research data, one might hypothesize that the nature of the perceived competence–physical activity relationship in the obese is similar to that for the normal weight child. However, obese children face the added complications of greater body weight (a negative predictor of activity in its own right) and a stigmatizing social environment that further discourages physical activity participation. The following section of the chapter outlines how constructs related to perceived competence can be incorporated to improve the design and implementation of physical activity programmes for obese children.

Recommendations for design and delivery of physical activity interventions

It is apparent that perceived competence plays an important role in obese children's participation in physical activity. The identification and subsequent exploitation of key mechanisms involved in the motivation of obese children to participate in physical activity and exercise, in the short and long term, is a substantive challenge. Using a blend of the key motivational theories outlined above, the constructs of age, significant others, motivational climate and dispositional goal orientation, perceived control, and task value will be reviewed briefly with practical recommendations for healthcare professionals involved in the design and delivery of interventions for the overweight or obese child.

Age

Sources used by children to formulate their perceptions of competence follow a developmental pattern based on age and other constructs. Therefore, it is necessary to adjust methods utilized to improve perceptions of competence and self-esteem according to the developmental status of the client group. For example, the goal orientation, conception of ability, perceived competence and the salient sources of feedback a child uses differ throughout the childhood years, with varying impacts on motivation. It is generally agreed that as children progress through the school system they shift from a task-oriented to an ego-oriented goal (Digelidis *et al.*, 2003; Xiang and Lee, 1998). Wigfield *et al.* (1997) established that both competence beliefs and beliefs about the usefulness and importance of different activities decline from early childhood to middle adolescence.

Nicholls, Jagacinski and Miller (1986) detailed the differentiation of concepts of ability, difficulty and effort with age. As children progress from early to middle childhood, their perceptions of difficulty shift from egocentric at ages 2–4, through objective (age 4/5–6), to normative at 6–7 years. The concept of effort at the early ages (4–5/6) is equated with ability. At age 7–9 equal effort is expected to lead to equal outcomes. Ability and effort only start to become differentiated at 9–10 years whereas complete differentiation and ability conceived as capacity is reached at 10–11/12 years. This sequence was also substantiated by Xiang and Lee (1998) and Lee, Carter and Xiang (1995).

Another feature of development is the tendency for children's accuracy of self-appraisal to increase and perceptions of competence to decrease. Digelidis and Papaioannou (1999) supported this hypothesis, finding that senior high school students had lower scores on perceived athletic ability than junior high and elementary school students. Horn and Weiss (1991) and Horn and Harris (1996) supported these findings, while suggesting that children may overestimate their skills when asked to rate general competence in a certain domain but may be more realistic and more accurate when asked to rate their competence in regard to specific skills.

Another distinguishing factor associated with age and stage of development is the preference for sources of physical competence information. Weiss, Ebbeck and Horn (1997) found that younger children (8–9 years) rated the use of parental evaluation comparatively higher and social comparison and evaluation lower than older children (10–13 years). According to the review by Horn and Harris (1996) children at a young age primarily use task accomplishment to assess their competence with a secondary source being feedback from significant adults. At this age, the feedback children receive is taken at face value and overrides other competence information such as peer comparison. Peer comparison begins to be used at approximately 7–8 years of age and increases steadily in importance until it is the most important source by the age of 12. Conversely, feedback from parents gradually decreases in importance over the same age range while feedback from the coach or teacher remains important to the child. Interestingly, children in the older years of this age range may no longer take adult feedback at face value and begin to evaluate it relative to other sources of competence information. This information is particularly relevant when considering the impact significant others have on a child's perception of competence and motivation to participate in physical activity.

During early childhood (3–6 years) the enhancement of competence can stem from multiple opportunities for children to demonstrate mastery or task accomplishment experiences (Horn and Harris, 1996). Feedback from parents/teachers/health professionals should encompass positive feedback that is contingent on task completion as opposed to peer comparison or task criteria. This will reinforce task goal orientation in the child with performance being judged by effort exerted, rather than comparison with the performance of peers.

During middle childhood (7–12 years), Craig, Goldberg and Dietz (1996) suggest that enabling each child to participate in physical activities in which they experience a sense of 'being good at it' presents an important way to increase perceived behavioural control in relation to physical activity. Thus, the emphasis should be on providing activities that are suitable to the physical maturity and ability of the child, thereby maximizing the chance that all children achieve some degree of task success. Adults working with children in this setting should aim to decrease the emphasis on peer comparison to evaluate performance and encourage the use of self-comparison. This is especially important for the obese; many of whom may not have succeeded during sport and physical activity in comparison with peers, resulting in low perceptions of competence. Obese children can be taught to evaluate their performance in terms of the personal improvements made in the development of skills. Consistent with such an approach, the teacher/coach/parent/health professional must provide children with appropriate and contingent performance feedback that encourages emphasis on skill technique as opposed to performance outcome.

In the early and middle childhood years, exercise interventions for the overweight and obese should initially be conducted in settings that do not facilitate comparison with children of normal weight. For example, a clinical weight management setting in which all staff are sympathetic to the individual needs of children would be an ideal scenario. Activities designed to provide each child with a sense of mastery/accomplishment over the task should be appropriate to the age and ability of the individuals. A task goal orientation should be emphasized by reinforcing achievement of self-set goals and improvements in technique. Feedback to children should be situation-appropriate and always emphasize that success stems from internally controllable factors. Wherever possible, parents should be involved in the treatment programme and provided with knowledge and understanding necessary to assist in fostering a positive attitude towards physical activity in their child. The scenario described above does exist, in the form of a residential childhood obesity camp. The aim of the camp is to provide a safe, supportive environment in which overweight and obese children could reduce their body mass and improve their health and well-being whilst having fun. In addition, the child-centred approach of the programme is focused on providing children with positive experiences and appropriate strategies that could continue when they return home. The daily schedule of physical activity combines a range of structured fun-type, skill-based activities. Evidence shows that the camp is successful at improving self-efficacy and general self perceptions (Gately *et al.*, 2005; Walker *et al.*, 2003), resulting in general psychological benefit (Barton *et al.*, 2004). Interestingly, a greater psychological benefit is associated with greater weight loss (Walker *et al.*, 2003).

Significant adults are the primary source of information for the development of perceived competence information in the middle to late childhood years (7–12 years) (Boyd and Hrycaiko, 1997). As a result it may be reasonable to conclude that, in this age range, children may be more receptive to interventions aimed at increasing the perceptions of competence as adult sources are commonly used for competence information. This is an important area of future research. Boyd and Hrycaiko (1997) found that pre-adolescents aged 9–10 years experienced the greatest gain in self-esteem after a physical activity intervention compared to those in early and middle adolescence. Braet, Mervielde and Vandereycken (1997) suggest that weight becomes a more important determinant of self-esteem in children with increasing age as the use of peer evaluation becomes more dominant in their lives. Thus, during the pre-adolescent years, interventions could capitalize on the lack of negative perceptions of self-esteem in obese young children as proposed by Kaplan and Wadden (1986).

Influence of significant others

The influence of significant others can shape a child's perception of competence as well as the motivational orientation and the child's perceptions of control (Weiss, 1987). The influence of significant others differs by age and developmental stage as previously mentioned. Brustad (1996) claimed that, up to the age of 10, parental influences have the most impact on the development of children's self-concept for a number of reasons. First, a large proportion of the child's time is spent within the context of the family; second, children have not developed the necessary social skills to establish social relationships outside the family; and third, children at this age rely heavily on feedback from parents and other adults in assessing personal competency. This high level of reliance on the family as a source of competence information and also social support should not be overlooked in the design of intervention programmes to assist in motivating young children to exercise. Evidence suggests that parents can have a positive influence by instilling perceptions of competence in their children (Biddle and Goudas, 1996; Brustad, 1993, 1996; McCullagh *et al.*, 1993; Welk, Wood and Morss, 2003).

Evidence abounds to support the key role of parents in children's perceived physical competence (McElroy, 2002) and physical activity behaviour (Dempsey, Kimiecik and Horn, 1993; Welk, Wood and Morss, 2003; Xiang, McBride and Bruene, 2003). Davison and Birch (2001) researched this relationship including the factor of weight status and found that parental concern about child weight status was associated with lower perceived physical ability on the part of the child. In some families with overweight children, parents may not be willing to encourage their children to participate in activity as they perceive that their child is not capable of achieving success because of their level of overweight. Over time this attitude may compound the child's weight problem. Parents who have realistic expectations, who provide support and encouragement for their children's efforts, and who rarely respond with negative evaluation, are more likely to have children who enjoy physical activity participation.

Although it is difficult to control the reactions and attitudes of peers, it is important for parents, teachers, coaches and health professionals to understand how peer interactions influence the perceptions of competence in obese children. A study by Weiss and Duncan (1992) reported on a strong association between physical competence and peer acceptance, concluding that a child's actual and perceived competence is strongly related to success in peer relations and perceived acceptance by the peer group. Conversely, Rose, Larkin and Berger (1997) found that failure in the movement setting has consequences for self-perception that may extend into the other domains of self-concept. Also, Braet, Mervielde and Vandereycken (1997) suggested that children with low perceived competence in the physical domain tend also to view themselves that way in social and self-worth. A logical conclusion might be that increases in physical competence could lead to improvements in perceptions of competence in other areas. However, this needs to be explored in further research. Similarly, further research is warranted to determine whether peer relations can directly or indirectly influence participation behaviour through self-perceptions, affect and general self-worth.

In recognition of the interrelatedness of the physical and social competence domains, the paediatric health professional must consider the social environment in which planned interventions are to occur and design such interventions to create an environment consistent with strengthening the positive self-concept. In the privacy of an obesity clinic with other children of similar size, shape and physical ability, the overweight child may feel more comfortable and competent than in a school-based setting where other more physically competent children dominate. Involving one or both parents in planning the physical activity prescription will offer the opportunity for the health professional to emphasize for the parent the importance of their role in communicating success expectations to their child to increase perceptions of competence.

Motivational climate and goal orientations

Based on the work of Nicholls and Miller (1984), ego and task goal orientations explain differences in perceptions of competence and both have different tendencies and characteristics in relation to persistence with physical activity. Compared to ego involvement, in which one's intrinsic interest in the task and desire to engage in it for its own sake is reduced (Duda, 1987), task orientation is more conducive to continuous participation in sport or physical activity. The two motivational climates (mastery- and performance-oriented) emphasize the task and ego goals respectively.

Fox *et al.* (1994) found that a group of children with high task orientation and low ego orientation had the lowest number of children with low perceived competence. Children with low perceived competence were less likely to choose task-oriented goals or, alternatively, high task orientation was more likely to encourage positive perceptions of competence. Further research is warranted, as there has been a failure to demonstrate in which direction causality exists. Xiang and Lee (1998) used a similar method to Fox *et al.* (1994) and concluded that those students who held a task orientation were more likely to hold an undifferentiated view of ability, meaning that they equated ability with effort. The implications of this finding for health professionals working with the obese is that, by creating a task-orientated environment in which ability is judged in a self-referenced manner, the professional is able to help individuals believe that ability can be developed with effort and therefore create a more self-motivated group of individuals.

The findings of Treasure (1997) are consistent with those of Fox *et al.* (1994) and Xiang and Lee (1998). Children who perceived a high mastery-/moderate performance-oriented climate held high perceptions of ability and believed effort (as opposed to external factors) to be the cause of success. Results of this study were also congruent with Ebbeck and Weiss (1998), who demonstrated that a high mastery/moderate performance climate was positively related to improved affective responses. Williams and Gill (1995) provided further support for the concept that perceived competence is related to a task orientation, establishing that a task goal orientation fosters children's perceptions of competence. Feelings of perceived competence lead to greater intrinsic interest, which in turn leads to greater effort. The work of Stephens (1998) substantiated these conclusions and reported that task orientation was significantly and positively related to perceived ability, enjoyment and value experienced through the sport of soccer.

Two studies have reported on successful changes to the motivational climate and subsequent increase in task orientation of students with resultant improved attitudes towards exercise (Digelidis and Papaioannou, 1999; Digelidis *et al.*, 2003). These findings suggest that when encouraging obese children to participate in activity the creation of a task-oriented motivational climate is most beneficial for perception of competence. Notably, Southall *et al.* (2004) successfully increased both the motor development and the perceived competence of a small group of overweight and obese children using a mastery motivational environment. Nine months after baseline, motor development and perceived competence were still significantly higher than at the start of the intervention. Further research in larger subject groups is required to substantiate these results, and the long-term effect this could have on physical activity participation and indicators of obesity. The environment can be structured to increase the child's task orientation by rewarding the achievement of self-determined goals that are not comparatively based. Reinforcement of form or technique is superior to a concentration on performance outcome in learning motor skills. Similarly, emphasizing self-comparison as a source of competence information, and the reinforcement of effort, persistence and a positive attitude towards exercise, are valuable (Weiss and Ebbeck, 1996). Xiang and Lee (1998) proposed that professionals should also encourage children to maintain or develop an undifferentiated conception of ability, whereby if one is trying hard they are considered successful. Practical strategies that can be utilized to foster better outcomes in this area include defining success in terms of mastering the task rather than outperforming others, emphasizing learning processes and participation, recognizing individual accomplishments, presenting tasks in an interesting manner, and evaluating on the basis of mastery and skill development rather than ability. For further details of how motivational climate can be adjusted to enhance motivation, readers are encouraged to refer to the work of Treasure and Roberts (1995) and Digelidis *et al.* (2003).

Perceptions of control

The Self-Determination Theory proposes that feelings of intrinsic motivation are maximized when an individual feels competent and in control of their participation (Ryan and Deci, 2002). Brunel (1999) adopted the framework of the Achievement Goal Theory and Self-Determination Theory to investigate the role of dispositional goal orientation and motivational climate in predicting intrinsic and extrinsic motivations and amotivation. Motivations were measured using the self-determination continuum, which describes the motivational constructs of amotivation, extrinsic and intrinsic motivation in terms of the individual's sense of self-determination when adopting a particular motivation. Findings revealed that perceptions of a mastery-oriented climate are related to the dimensions of intrinsic motivation which lie at the more self-determined end of the continuum. Hassandra, Goudas and Chroni (2003) also found that students with high intrinsic motivation scores felt more self-determined. The direction of causality in both studies was undetermined, but one could argue for the development of a mastery motivational climate in settings where children engage in physical activity.

Vlachopoulos and Biddle (1996) and Vlachopoulos, Biddle and Fox (1997) investigated the concepts of goal orientations, perceived sport competence, attributions and affect states in children's physical education. Their findings revealed that perceived competence was significantly correlated with perceived success which was then significantly correlated with the dimensions of causality and personal control. Notably, perceptions of success had a positive direct effect on positive affect variables. It has been theorized that this effect contributes to the likelihood of involvement in sport and exercise in adulthood. It was also revealed that only internal attributions for success were found to predict positive achievement-related affect (Haywood, 1991).

Spray and Wang (2001) found a relationship between perceived competence and feelings of self-determination such that students with lower perceptions of their own competence held less autonomous reasons for behaviour, whereas those with higher perceptions of competence felt more autonomous about their behaviour. It is not possible to determine the causal pathway from these data; however, one could infer that assisting students to make internal attributions for their behaviour as undertaken by Sinnott and Biddle (1998) could improve their perceptions of competence and thus intrinsic motivation.

There also seems to be some consensus in the literature that a task orientation is associated with internal attributions for success (Brunel, 1999; Cury *et al.*, 1997; Duda *et al.*, 1992; Spray and Wang, 2001; Vlachopoulos and Biddle, 1996; Vlachopoulos, Biddle and Fox, 1997; Walling and Duda, 1995), which emphasizes again the need to support children in the weight management setting to develop a task orientation in order to foster improved perceptions of competence and thus increase intrinsic motivation.

Task value

Ferguson *et al.* (1989) found the perceived benefits of exercise correlated significantly with intention to exercise in a group of preadolescents. These findings agreed with Dempsey, Kimiecik and Horn (1993), who examined parents' and children's belief systems about moderate to vigorous physical activity (MVPA) using the expectancy–value model. They found that parents' perception of their children's physical competence was a significant predictor of their child's MVPA, while children's positive expectancies about MVPA and task orientation were also a significant predictor of MVPA participation after controlling for gender.

Cury *et al.* (1997) identified that those youngsters who perceived themselves as incompetent at a task assigned less value to that task than those who had a high perceived ability, and those who had low perceived ability invested less in the task. This is an important factor to consider when encouraging the overweight and obese population to be more active. Shapiro and Ulrich (2002) suggest that, to enhance motivation, teachers, parents and significant others should take the opportunity to highlight the importance and usefulness of exercise and physical activity and create new and exciting activities for learning which enable enjoyment of physical activity to be experienced. It is also important to connect physical activity in the school, home or other settings with benefits in other domains of life, thereby increasing the perceived value of physical activity in its own right.

Conclusions

A common misconception is that all obese children need the same advice: namely to be encouraged to move. However, encouragement needs to be matched with the provision of opportunity and formal recognition of the many idiosyncrasies commonly seen in obese children. For example, many obese children are regularly confronted with situations that may be stigmatizing and that may contribute to decreases in self-esteem. This may be especially poignant if the stigmatizing situation occurs in the context of sport or physical activity and leads to a decrease in motivation to exercise. Obese children are confronted with a series of physical and psychological barriers that influence their perceived competence to be physically active. By being aware that perceived competence plays an important role in obese children's participation in physical activity and implementing the recommendations proposed in this chapter, teachers and health professionals can take positive steps to contribute a more positive self-concept in these children and, thus, a more holistic approach to the treatment of childhood obesity.

References

Baranowski, T., Mendlein, J., Resnicow, K., Frank, E., Webber Cullen, K. and Baranowski, J. (2000) 'Physical activity and nutrition in children and youth: an overview of obesity prevention', *Preventive Medicine*, 31: S1–10.

Barton, S.B., Walker, L.L.M., Lambert, G., Gately, P.J. and Hill, A.J. (2004) 'Cognitive changes in obese adolescents losing weight', *Obesity Research*, 12: 313–19.

Biddle, S. and Goudas, M. (1996) 'Analysis of children's physical activity and its association with adult encouragement and social cognitive variables', *Journal of School Health*, 66: 75–8.

Boyd, K.R. and Hrycaiko, D.W. (1997) 'The effect of a physical activity intervention package on the self-esteem of pre-adolescent and adolescent females', *Adolescence*, 32: 693–708.

Braet, C., Mervielde, I. and Vandereycken, W. (1997) 'Psychological aspects of childhood obesity: a controlled study in a clinical and non-clinical sample', *Journal of Pediatric Psychology*, 22: 59–71.

Brownell, K.D. (1995) 'Exercise and obesity treatment: psychological aspects', *International Journal of Obesity and Related Metabolic Disorders*, 19: S122–5.

Brunel, P.C. (1999) 'Relationship between achievement goal orientations and perceived motivational climate on intrinsic motivation', *Scandinavian Journal of Medicine and Science in Sports*, 9: 365–74.

Brustad, R.J. (1993) 'Who will go out and play? Parental and psychological influences on children's attraction to physical activity', *Pediatric Exercise Science*, 5: 210–23.

Brustad, R.J. (1996) 'Parental and peer influence on children's psychological development through sport', in F.L. Smoll, R.E. Smith (eds) *Children and Youth in Sport: A Biopsychosocial Perspective*, Madison, WI: Brown and Benchmark, pp. 112–24.

Causgrove Dunn, J. (2000) 'Goal orientations, perceptions of the motivational climate, and perceived competence of children with movement difficulties', *Adapted Physical Activity Quarterly*, 17: 1–19.

Craig, S., Goldberg, J. and Dietz, W. (1996) 'Psychosocial correlates of physical activity among fifth and eighth graders', *Preventative Medicine*, 25: 506–13.

Cury, F., Biddle, S., Sarrazin, P. and Famose, J.P. (1997) 'Achievement goals and perceived ability predict investment in learning a sport task', *British Journal of Educational Psychology*, 67: 39–43; 293–309.

Davies, P.S.W., Gregory, J. and White, A. (1995) 'Physical activity and body fatness in pre-school children', *International Journal of Obesity and Related Metabolic Disorders*, 19: 6–10.

Davison, K.K. and Birch, L.L. (2001) 'Weight status, parent reaction, and self-concept in five-year-old girls', *Pediatrics*, 107: 46–53.

Deci, E.L. and Ryan, R.M. (1985) *Intrinsic Motivation and Self-Determination in Human Behavior*, New York: Plenum.

Dempsey, J.M., Kimiecik, J.C. and Horn, T.S. (1993) 'Parental influence on children's moderate to vigorous physical activity participation: an expectancy–value approach', *Pediatric Exercise Science*, 5: 151–67.

Digelidis, N. and Papaioannou, A. (1999) 'Age-group differences in intrinsic motivation, goal orientations and perceptions of athletic competence, physical appearance and motivational climate in Greek physical education', *Scandinavian Journal of Medicine and Science in Sports*, 9: 375–81.

Digelidis, N., Papaioannou, A., Laparidis, K. and Christodoulidis, T. (2003) 'A one year intervention in 7th grade physical education classes aiming to change motivational climate and attitudes towards exercise', *Psychology of Sport and Exercise*, 4: 195–210.

Duda, J.L. (1987) 'Toward a developmental theory of children's motivation in sport', *Journal of Sport Psychology*, 9: 130–45.

Duda, J.L., Fox, K.R., Biddle, S.J. and Armstrong, N. (1992) 'Children's achievement goals and beliefs about success in sport', *British Journal of Educational Psychology*, 62: 313–23.

Ebbeck, V. and Weiss, M.R. (1998) 'Determinants of children's self-esteem: an examination of perceived competence and affect in sport', *Pediatric Exercise Science*, 10: 285–98.

Eccles (Parsons), J.S., Adler, T.F., Futterman, R., Goff, S.B., Kaczala, C.M., Meece, J.L. and Midgley, C. (1983) 'Expectancies, values and academic behaviours', in J.T. Spence (ed.) *Achievement and Achievement Motivation*, San Francisco, CA: Freeman, pp. 75–146.

Ekkekakis, P., Hall, E. and Petrizzello, S. (2005) 'Variation and homogeneity in affective responses to physical activity of varying intensities: an alternative perspective on dose-response based on evolutionary considerations', *Journal of Sports Science*, 23: 477–500.

Ekkekakis, P. and Lind, E. (2006) 'Exercise does not feel the same when you are overweight: the impact of self-selected and imposed intensity on affect and exertion', *International Journal of Obesity and Related Metabolic Disorders*, 3: 652–60.

Elliott, M.A., Copperman, N.M. and Jacobson, M.S. (2004) 'Pediatric obesity prevention and management', *Minerva Pediatrica*, 56: 265–76.

Epstein, L.H., Paluch, R.A., Coleman, K.J., Vito, D. and Anderson, K. (1996) 'Determinants of physical activity in obese children assessed by accelerometer and self-report', *Medicine and Science in Sports and Exercise*, 28: 1157–64.

Ferguson, K., Yesalis, C., Pomrehn, P. and Kirkpatrick, M. (1989) 'Attitudes, knowledge, and beliefs as predictors of exercise intent and behavior in schoolchildren', *Journal of School Health*, 59: 112–15.

Flodmark, C.E., Lissau, I., Moreno, L.A., Pietrobelli, A. and Widhalm, K. (2004) 'New insights into the field of children and adolescents' obesity: the European perspective', *International Journal of Obesity and Related Metabolic Disorders*, 28: 1189–96.

Fox, K., Goudas, M., Biddle, S., Duda, J.L. and Armstrong, N. (1994) 'Children's task and ego goal profiles in sport', *British Journal of Educational Psychology*, 64: 253–61.

Gately, P.J., Cooke, C.B., Barth, J.H., Bewick, B.M., Radley, D. and Hill, A.J. (2005) 'Children's residential weight loss programs can work: a prospective cohort study of short-term outcomes for overweight and obese children', *Pediatrics*, 116: 73–7.

Harter, S. (1981) 'A model of mastery motivation in children: individual differences and developmental change', in W. A. Collins (ed.) *The Minnesota Symposium on Child Psychology. Aspects of the Development of Competence*, Vol. 14, Hillsdale, NJ: Lawrence Erlbaum Associates: pp. 215–55.

Harter, S. (1990) 'Processes underlying adolescent self-concept formation', in R. Montmayer, G. R. Adams, T. P. Gullotta (eds) *Advances in Adolescent Development, Vol. 2: From Childhood to Adolescence – A Transition Period*, London: Sage, pp. 352–87.

Harter, S. and Connell, J.P. (1984) 'A model of children's achievement and related self-perceptions of competence, control, and motivational orientation', in J. Nicholls (ed.), *Advances in Motivation and Achievement, Vol. 3: The Development of Achievement Motivation*, Greenwich, CT: JAI Press, pp. 219–50.

Hassandra, M., Goudas, M. and Chroni, S. (2003) 'Examining factors associated with intrinsic motivation in physical education: a qualitative approach', *Psychology of Sport and Exercise*, 4: 211–23.

Haywood, K.M. (1991) 'The role of physical education in the development of active lifestyles', *Research Quarterly for Exercise and Sport*, 62: 151–6.

Hills, A.P. (1994) 'Locomotor characteristics of obese children', in A.P. Hills, M.L. Wahl-qvist (eds) *Exercise and Obesity*, London: Smith Gordon, pp. 141–50.

Hills, A. (1998) 'Scholastic and intellectual development and sports', in K. Chan and L. Micheli (eds) *Sports and Children*, Hong Kong: Williams and Wilkins, pp. 76–90.

Horn, T.S. and Harris, A. (1996) 'Perceived competence in young athletes: research findings and recommendations for coaches and parents', in F.L. Smoll, R.E. Smith (eds) *Children and Youth in Sport: A Biopsychosocial Perspective*, Madison, WI: Brown and Benchmark, pp. 309–29.

Horn, T.S. and Weiss, M.R. (1991) 'A developmental analysis of children's self-ability judgments in the physical domain', *Pediatric Exercise Science*, 3: 310–26.

Kaplan, K.M. and Wadden, T.A. (1986) 'Childhood obesity and self-esteem', *Journal of Pediatrics*, 109: 367–70.

Korsch, B. (1986) 'Childhood obesity', *Journal of Pediatrics*, 109: 229–300.

Lee, A.M., Carter, J.A. and Xiang, P. (1995) 'Children's conceptions of ability in physical education', *Journal of Teaching in Physical Education*, 14: 384–93.

McCullagh, P., Matzkanin, K.T., Shaw, S.D. and Maldonado, M. (1993) 'Motivation for participation in physical activity: a comparison of parent–child perceived competencies and participation motives', *Pediatric Exercise Science*, 5: 224–33.

McElroy, M. (2002) *Resistance to Exercise: A Social Analysis of Inactivity*, Champaign, IL: Human Kinetics.

Mulvihill, A., Rivers, K. and Aggleton, P. (2000) *Physical Activity 'At Our Time': Qualitative Research among Young People Aged 5 to 15 Years and Parents*, London: Health Education Authority.

Myers, A. and Rosen, J.C. (1999) 'Obesity stigmatization and coping: relation to mental health symptoms, body image, and self-esteem', *International Journal of Obesity and Related Metabolic Disorders*, 23: 221–30.

Neumark-Sztainer, D., Story, M. and Faibisch, L. (1998) 'Perceived stigmatization among overweight African-American and Caucasian adolescent girls', *Journal of Adolescent Health*, 23: 264–70.

Nicholls, J.G. (1989) *The Competitive Ethos and Democratic Education*, Cambridge, MA: Harvard University Press.

Nicholls, J.G. and Miller, A.T. (1984) 'Development and its discontents: the differentiation of the concept of ability', in J. Nicholls (ed.) *Advances in Motivation and Achievement, Vol. 3: The Development of Achievement Motivation*, Greenwich, CT: JAI Press, pp. 185–218.

Nicholls, J.G., Jagacinski, C.M. and Miller, A.T. (1986) 'Conceptions of ability in children and adults', in R. Schwarzer (ed.) *Self-related Cognitions in Anxiety and Motivation*, Hillsdale, NJ: Erlbaum, pp. 265–84.

Parízková, J., Hainer, V., Stich, V., Kunesova, M. and Ksantini, M. (1994) 'Physiological capabilities of obese individuals and implications for exercise', in A.P. Hills, M.L. Wahl-qvist (eds) *Exercise and Obesity*, London: Smith Gordon, pp. 131–40.

Phillips, R.G. and Hill, A.J. (1998) 'Fat, plain, but not friendless: self-esteem and peer acceptance of obese pre-adolescent girls', *International Journal of Obesity and Related Metabolic Disorders*, 22: 287–93.

Pierce, J.W. and Wardle, J. (1993) 'Self-esteem, parental appraisal and body size in children', *Child Psychology and Psychiatry*, 34: 1125–36.

Roberts, G.C., Kleiber, D.A. and Duda, J.L. (1981) 'An analysis of motivation in children's sport: the role of percieved competence in participation', *Journal of Sport Psychology*, 3: 206–16.

Rose, B., Larkin, D. and Berger, B. (1997) 'Coordination and gender influences on the perceived competence of children', *Adapted Physical Activity Quarterly*, 14: 210–21.

Rowland, T.W. (2004) 'The childhood obesity epidemic: putting the dynamics into thermodynamics', *Pediatric Exercise Science*, 16: 87–93.

Ryan, R.M. and Deci, E.L. (2002) 'Overview of self-determination theory: an organismic-dialectical perspective', in E.L. Deci, R.M. Ryan (eds) *Handbook of Self-Determination Research*, Rochester, NY: University of Rochester Press, pp. 3–33.

Shapiro, D.R. and Ulrich, D.A. (2002) 'Expectancies, values, and perceptions of physical competence of children with and without learning disabilities', *Adapted Physical Activity Quarterly*, 19: 318–33.

Sinnott, K. and Biddle, S. (1998) 'Changes in attributions, perceptions of success and intrinsic motivation after attribution retraining in children's sport', *International Journal of Adolescence and Youth*, 7: 137–44.

Solmon, M.A., Lee, A.M., Belcher, D., Harrison, L., Jr and Wells, L. (2003) 'Beliefs about gender appropriateness, ability, and competence in physical activity', *Journal of Teaching in Physical Education*, 22: 261–79.

Southall, J.E., Okely, A.D. and Steele, J.R. (2004) 'Actual and perceived physical competence in overweight and non-overweight children', *Pediatric Exercise Science*, 16: 15–25.

Spray, C.M. and Wang, C.K. (2001) 'Goal orientations, self-determination and pupils' discipline in physical education', *Journal of Sports Sciences*, 19: 903–13.

Steinbeck, K.S. (2001) 'The importance of physical activity in the prevention of overweight and obesity in childhood: a review and an opinion', *Obesity Reviews*, 2: 117–30.

Stephens, D.E. (1998) 'The relationship of goal orientation and perceived ability to enjoyment and value in youth sport', *Pediatric Exercise Science*, 10: 236–47.

Stunkard, A.J. (1996) 'Current views on obesity', *American Journal of Medicine*, 100: 230–6.

Taylor, W.C. and Sallis, J.F. (1997) 'Determinants of physical activity in children', in A.P. Simopoulus, K.N. Pavlou (eds) *Nutrition and Fitness: Metabolic and Behavioural Aspects in Health and Disease, Vol. 82*, Basel: Karger, pp. 159–67.

Theeboom, M., De Knop, P. and Weiss, M.R. (1995) 'Motivational climate, psychological responses, and motor skill development in children's sport: a field-based intervention study', *Journal of Sport and Exercise Psychology*, 17: 294–311.

Treasure, D.C. (1997) 'Perceptions of the motivational climate and elementary school children's cognitive and affective response', *Journal of Sport and Exercise Psychology*, 19: 278–90.

Treasure, D.C. and Roberts, G.C. (1995) 'Applications of achievement goal theory to physical education: implications for enhancing motivation', *Quest*, 47: 475–89.

Vlachopoulos, S. and Biddle, S. (1996) 'A social-cognitive investigation into the mechanisms of affect generation in children's physical activity', *Journal of Sport and Exercise Psychology*, 18: 174–93.

Vlachopoulos, S., Biddle, S. and Fox, K. (1997) 'Determinants of emotion in children's physical activity: a test of goal perspectives and attribution theories', *Pediatric Exercise Science*, 9: 65–79.

Walker, L.M., Gately, P.J., Bewick, B.M. and Hill, A.J. (2003) 'Children's weight loss camps: psychological benefit or jeopardy?', *International Journal of Obesity and Related Metabolic Disorders*, 27: 748–54.

Walling, M.D. and Duda, J.L. (1995) 'Goals and their associations with beliefs about success in and perceptions of the purposes of physical education', *Journal of Teaching in Physical Education*, 14: 140–56.

Weiner, B. (1986) *An Attributional Theory of Motivation and Emotion*, New York: Springer-Verlag.

Weiss, M.R. (1987) 'Self-esteem and achievement in children's sport and physical activity', in D. Gould, M.R. Weiss (eds) *Advances in Pediatric Sport Sciences, Vol. 2: Behavioral Issues*, Champaign, IL: Human Kinetics, pp. 87–119.

Weiss, M.R. and Duncan, S.C. (1992) 'The relationship between physical competence and peer acceptance in the context of children's sport participation', *Journal of Sport and Exercise Psychology*, 14: 177–91.

Weiss, M.K. and Ebbeck, V. (1996) 'Self-esteem and perceptions of competence in youth sports: theory, research and enhancement strategies', in O. Bar-Or (ed.) *The Child and Adolescent Athlete: Vol. 6 of the Encyclopedia of Sports Medicine*, Oxford: Blackwell Science, pp. 364–82.

Weiss, M.R., Ebbeck, V. and Horn, T.S. (1997) 'Children's self-perceptions and sources of physical competence information: a cluster analysis', *Journal of Sport and Exercise Psychology*, 19: 52–70.

Welk, G.J., Wood, K. and Morss, G. (2003) 'Parental influences on physical activity in children: an exploration of potential mechanisms', *Pediatric Exercise Science*, 15: 19–33.

Wigfield, A., Eccles, J.S., Yoon, K.S., Harold, R.D., Arbreton, A.J.A., Freedman-Doan, C. and Blumenfeld, P.C. (1997) 'Change in children's competence beliefs and subjective task values across the elementary school years: a 3-year study', *Journal of Educational Psychology*, 89: 451–69.

Williams, L. and Gill, D. (1995) 'The role of perceived competence in the motivation of physical activity', *Journal of Sport and Exercise Psychology*, 17: 363–78.

Xiang, P. and Lee, A. (1998) 'The development of self-perceptions of ability and achievement goals and their relations in physical education', *Research Quarterly for Exercise and Sport*, 69: 231–41.

Xiang, P., McBride, R. and Bruene, A. (2003) 'Relations of parents' beliefs to children's motivation in an elementary physical education running program', *Journal of Teaching in Physical Education*, 22: 410–25.

7 Psychosocial aspects of childhood obesity

S.M. Byrne and M. La Puma

Introduction

Whereas the physical health risks of childhood obesity have been widely documented, much less research has focused on the social and psychological factors that appear to be associated with excess weight in childhood. Little is known about whether or not these psychosocial factors are risk factors for, or primarily consequences of, childhood obesity. Research focusing on the psychosocial aspects of childhood obesity is crucial for two main reasons: first because psychosocial problems (including problems such as teasing and bullying, low self-esteem, depression and eating disorders) are likely to have more impact on the lives of more obese children than any of the other adverse consequences associated with obesity; second because, although biological factors (such as genetic vulnerability) are likely to exert an important influence upon the development and persistence of obesity, if psychosocial factors also play an important role, they may be more amenable to modification.

This chapter will outline the social and psychological factors that research has suggested may be associated with childhood obesity. We will focus on those factors that have either been implicated in the development of obesity or have been identified as resulting from overweight or obesity in childhood. In many cases it is not yet clear whether the factors that we describe below are precursors of obesity, consequences of obesity or both.

Socioeconomic status

In 1989, Sobal and Stunkard published a comprehensive review of the literature that had examined the relationship between social class and obesity. Among adults, the data showed that in developed countries there is a strong inverse relationship between socioeconomic status (SES) and obesity in women (although not in men), with a higher proportion of obese women coming from the lower social classes. By contrast, in developing countries, there was a strong positive relationship between SES and obesity in women, men and children.

relationship between SES and obesity in children in developed countries is less well established. Of the studies reviewed by Sobal and Stunkard (1989) that included children, 40 per cent found no relationship between SES and obesity, 40 per cent found an inverse relationship and 20 per cent found a positive relationship. However, since this review, studies have begun to document more consistently a clear inverse relationship between SES and obesity in children, particularly among girls. Surveys of Australian children and adolescents have also observed this relationship (Booth *et al.*, 1999).

A Danish longitudinal study that reported on a 10-year follow-up of 9- to 10-year-olds (Lissau and Sorensen, 1994) identified that some specific socioeconomic factors were inversely related to children's overweight in adulthood, including parental education and parental occupation. The study also found that a general atmosphere of neglect (poor parental support and poor cleanliness) was significantly positively related to overweight in adulthood. The most significant risk factor for overweight in adulthood was quality of housing in childhood, even after controlling for parental education and occupation. The data suggested that being brought up in a deprived area of the city increased the risk of being overweight by over three times that of being brought up in a more affluent area.

What might explain the relationship between SES and obesity in developed countries?

It is often suggested that the stresses of low SES may somehow contribute to the development of greater rates of obesity in children. Researchers have suggested that socially disadvantaged families may have low levels of nutritional knowledge and interest, poor overall nutrition and few opportunities for physical activity, although few studies have actually examined the eating behaviour and activity levels of low SES children. There may, however, be other explanations for the relationship between SES and obesity. For example, it may be that obesity promotes a reduction in SES. There is ample evidence of discrimination against obese individuals in areas such as educational, employment and housing opportunities. Studies in the United Kingdom and in the United States have shown that women who had been overweight since adolescence completed fewer years of school, earned significantly less, had higher rates of household poverty and were less likely to be married than their lean peers (Gortmaker *et al.*, 1993). A third explanation may be that obesity and low SES share causes that lead to both conditions.

Societal attitudes toward obesity and discrimination

It is well documented that modern western society highly values attractiveness and thinness, and stigmatizes obesity, particularly in women. This negative perception of obesity is widespread and intense, and means that obese people often face discrimination in education, work, social relationships and healthcare (Gortmaker *et al.*, 1993).

There seem to be two principal aspects of the stigma of obesity. In the first place, there is the stigmatization of bodily appearance. Obesity is a highly visible state, and physical appearance (particularly body shape) is one of the most important factors in how people judge one another. In the second place there is the stigmatization of character: the moral view that holds obese individuals personally responsible for their own state. Whereas the ideal body is associated with connotations of competence, success, self-control, self-worth and acceptance, the converse is that overweight individuals are often looked upon as indulgent, lazy, weak-willed and lacking in control.

A range of research over the last 40 years has suggested that these negative attitudes originate in childhood. For example, in a very early study, Richardson *et al.* (1961) presented a series of six drawings to a group of 10- to 11-year-old children. One of the drawings depicted a physically normal child, and the other five drawings represented children with various disabilities, one of which was overweight. The participants were asked to rate the drawings and rank them in order of preference. The children consistently preferred the drawing of the child with no handicap, and the overweight child was consistently ranked last (below drawings of a child on crutches, a child in a wheelchair, a child with a hand missing and a child with a facial disfigurement). In another early study using a different technique, Stafferi (1967) presented 6- to 10-year-old boys with full-body silhouettes of a thin, a muscular and a fat body figure. The children were asked to assign a number of adjectives to each silhouette. Almost invariably, the fat body shape was labelled 'lazy', 'stupid', 'sloppy', 'dirty', 'naughty', 'mean' and 'ugly'. Subsequent studies using a range of alternative stimulus materials (such as photographs, written descriptions and rating scales) to examine children's attitudes to overweight and obesity have produced identical results. For example, Hill and Silver (1995) showed silhouettes of slim and fat children to 188 nine-year-old girls and boys, and asked them to comment on the perceived health and fitness of the children depicted in the silhouettes. The fat figures were judged to be extremely unhealthy, unfit and extremely unlikely to eat healthily.

A number of methodological problems with studies of this nature have been noted, including the issue of generalizability of drawings to real-life people, the confounding of facial attractiveness, the use of ranking and forced choice methods of assessment, and a failure to check children's perception of the degree of overweight depicted in drawings or photographs. Nevertheless, the findings have been remarkably consistent in suggesting that even very young children appear to have accepted the prevalent stereotypes associated with overweight; a specific rejection of fatness is clear. The results of these and similar studies also suggest that, overall, girls are less accepting of their overweight peers than are boys, and that negative attitudes toward obesity are more likely to be voiced by those from a higher SES background (Hill and Silver, 1995).

What about overweight children's views?

Few studies have investigated whether overweight children's attitudes toward obesity differ from those of their healthy weight peers. Those studies that have been able to examine this issue have found few differences (Hill and Silver, 1995).

Although Hill and Silver (1995) did observe some moderating effects of body mass index (BMI) in their study of stereotyped perception (they noticed that the heaviest children judged all of the silhouettes – fat and thin – to be fitter than did the lighter children), overall the overweight children did share the extremely negative perception of the fat figures.

The influence of parents, families and peers on the development and consequences of obesity

Parents

Over the last three decades, several researchers have hypothesized about the role that parental influence may play in the development and persistence of childhood obesity. Bruch (1973) was the first to suggest that early-onset obesity may stem from unhelpful learning in infancy. She hypothesized that mothers who fail to differentiate their child's need for food from signals regarding other aversive states may feed their child indiscriminately. This may lead the child to confuse hunger with other internal sensations (such as sadness, boredom, discomfort), and if this persists it could contribute to overeating and overweight.

Other researchers have considered the relationship between parental weight and attitudes toward weight and shape, and their children's weight and eating habits. This relationship is likely to be a complex one. Links have frequently been made between the dieting behaviour of mothers and that of their preadolescent and adolescent daughters – dieting mothers tend to have dieting daughters. Direct comments to children about their weight (especially comments from mothers to daughters) have also been associated with increased dieting behaviour in children (Pike and Rodin, 1991). This is important because longitudinal studies have confirmed that dieting and other weight-reduction efforts in adolescence are more likely to result in significant weight gain than in weight loss over time (Stice *et al.*, 1999).

Another line of research has been based on the idea that parents will be especially controlling in areas of their children's development in which they perceive the child to be at risk, or in areas in which parents have a high personal investment (Constanzo and Woody, 1985). Thus, an obese parent, or a parent who is very concerned about their own weight and shape, may be particularly concerned about their child's eating habits and perceive their child as being at risk of obesity. Ironically, persistent parental attempts to regulate their child's food intake may, in fact, be counterproductive. Parental over-control of what and how much a child eats may deprive the child of opportunities to learn to control his/her own eating behaviour and place the child at increased risk for obesity (Constanzo and Woody, 1985). There is some evidence to support this hypothesis. For example, Johnson and Birch (1994) conducted a series of laboratory studies to test 3- to 5-year-old children's ability to adjust their food intake in response to changes in the caloric density of their diet. They found that the best predictor of this ability was parental control of the feeding situation. Parents who were more controlling (using bribes, threats and food rewards to control food intake) had children who showed less ability to regulate energy intake. 'Over-controlling' mothers were also more likely themselves to be dieting. Other studies have also found that using foods as rewards, or restricting preferred foods, increases children's preferences for these foods, and that prompting and rewarding food intake tends to override children's self-regulation of food intake and lead to overeating and overweight. There also appears to be a moderating effect of gender, with parents being more inclined to take an active role in controlling the food intake of their obese daughters than of their obese sons (Constanzo and Woody, 1985).

It is not clear, however, whether high levels of parental control over eating causes childhood obesity by interfering with a child's self-regulation of eating or it represents attempts to minimize weight gain in an already overweight child.

Family functioning

A small number of interview and questionnaire studies have raised the question of whether families with obese children may behave differently to families with no obese children. Various studies have found 'obese' families to be characterized by a range of potential problems, including a tendency to cover up and avoid facing problems, low 'cohesion', low independence, poor marital relationships, direct criticism of the obese child, differential handling of children in the family, low levels of expressiveness, and an undemocratic parenting style (Mendelson, White and Schliecker, 1995). However, it is clear that these characteristics are not evident in every 'obese' family (or even in many) and, overall, there is no good evidence to suggest that the families of obese children are any more 'dysfunctional' than families of healthy-weight children. Once again, studies in this area have not been able to disentangle cause and effect. Do dysfunctional families contribute to the development of obesity? Or are family problems a consequence of the child's obesity? The most likely scenario is both. For example, some family circumstances may fail to facilitate a child's self-regulation abilities and contribute to weight gain. On other hand, parents who want to help their overweight child may become over-controlling of their eating behaviour and this intrusiveness may be viewed negatively by their children.

Peers

During early adolescence the balance of children's social support begins to shift from parents to peers (although parental social support rarely becomes unimportant). The nature of peer relationships also begins to change during adolescence, from mainly companionship to loyalty and intimacy. Although this more intense form of peer support can provide a buffer against the negative effects of life stress, teasing and bullying by peers during adolescence can be extremely harmful, especially when the focus is on a sensitive personal feature such as weight or shape. Several studies have found an association between frequency of teasing during childhood and adolescence and body dissatisfaction, low self-esteem and eating disturbances (Grilo *et al.*, 1994). Moreover, teasing about weight shape in childhood has been identified as a significant risk factor for the development of full-blown eating disorders in adolescence (Fairburn *et al.*, 1997).

Weight-related teasing certainly appears to be a common experience among obese children and adolescents. For example, Wilfley *et al.* (1998) found that 81 per cent of obese children attending a weight loss camp reported having been teased or criticized about their weight and being at least moderately distressed by this teasing. There are few data on the extent, nature and severity of weight-related teasing and other forms of victimization among obese children, however, and far more information about the consequences of teasing for overweight/obese children is needed.

Psychological factors

Very little research has attempted to identify psychological factors that may predispose a child to obesity. A small number of studies have examined whether temperament characteristics in infancy may predict later obesity in children; however, it is not possible to generalize from these studies and further investigation in this area is required. Research into the psychological health of already obese children is also limited. Even in the adult literature, the relationship between obesity and psychological health remains unclear. Overall, research has tended to suggest that, despite the stigmatization of obesity and the associated discrimination, obesity is not associated with general psychological problems, and that the variation in psychological adjustment in obese samples is comparable to that found in the population at large (Friedman and Brownell, 1995). Several studies have documented few differences between obese and non-obese adults and adolescents in terms of scores on various measures of depression, anxiety, body image and self-esteem (Friedman and Brownell, 1995).

These studies, however, have generally used only one or two select unidimensional measures (such as the State–Trait Anxiety Inventory or the Rosenberg Self-Esteem Scale) to compare obese individuals with non-obese individuals. Research using broader measures, including diagnostic instruments and structured face-to-face interviews, has been able to detect significantly higher rates of depression and anxiety in obese than non-obese individuals, particularly among women and adolescent females (Carpenter *et al.*, 2000). Moreover, clinicians and researchers are beginning to recognize that the obese population is strikingly heterogeneous with respect to both its aetiology and its consequences (Friedman and Brownell, 1995). Thus, obesity may be associated with significant psychological problems in some individuals, mild problems in others, and none in others. Only a very small number of studies have begun to try to tease out the factors that might influence which obese individuals will be most vulnerable to developing psychological problems. These studies have suggested that, among obese subjects, being younger, female or more severely obese, or having had an early onset of obesity, is associated with a higher risk of psychological impairment (Mustillo *et al.*, 2003).

It is also possible that, although obesity may not lead directly to psychological problems, it may contribute indirectly to poor psychological health. In one of the few studies to examine the mental health of obese children, Hill, Draper and Stack (1994) found that poor mental health was not the inevitable consequence of even the most extreme obesity in children. However, low self-esteem and poor peer relationships, which were significantly associated with being overweight, were, in turn, found to be significant predictors of poor overall mental health. Thus obesity, through its relationship with low self-esteem and poor peer relationships, was indirectly linked with psychological health.

Some research has suggested that, although obese individuals may not differ from non-obese individuals with regard to scores on standard psychological tests or on general measures of psychopathology, they may suffer from specific psychological problems related to their obesity. Three psychological problems that appear to be specifically associated with obesity are body dissatisfaction, low self-esteem and binge eating. These aspects of psychological health with regard to obese children will be discussed in turn.

Body dissatisfaction

The term 'body dissatisfaction' is widely used to refer to the cognitive/affective aspects of body image, that is an individual's subjective evaluation of their body shape and weight. Body dissatisfaction is considered to be one of the most personal and psychologically distressing components of obesity. Within the obese population (as in the general population), body dissatisfaction probably occurs on a continuum ranging from mild feelings of unattractiveness to an extreme preoccupation with physical appearance that impairs day-to-day functioning. Among obese adults, body dissatisfaction is reported to occur most often in individuals with childhood-onset obesity, who have faced negative teasing about their weight and shape during childhood and adolescence from their family and/or their peers, and obese women generally report greater body dissatisfaction than do obese men (Grilo et al., 1994).

Many studies using well-validated measures have demonstrated that, compared with normal-weight adults, obese adults are more dissatisfied and preoccupied with their physical appearance, and avoid more social situations on account of their appearance (Sarwer, Wadden and Foster, 1998). A substantial proportion of obese women in particular report experiencing extreme embarrassment in social settings, camouflaging their appearance with clothing and avoiding looking at their body (Sarwer, Wadden and Foster, 1998).

In young people as well, there is a clear association between overweight and body dissatisfaction, especially among girls (Hill, Draper and Stack, 1994). This association is apparent by eight years of age and possibly earlier (Hill and Pallin, 1998). Many children and adolescents (again, particularly girls) express preferences for a slimmer figure, but there is a marked effect of actual weight, with studies showing that overweight children's desire to be thinner is almost unanimous (Hill, Draper and Stack, 1994). Whereas in adults body dissatisfaction has been found to be significantly associated with other psychological problems such as depressive symptoms and low self-esteem (Grilo *et al.*, 1994; Sarwer, Wadden and Foster, 1998), these links have not been investigated in obese children.

Low self-esteem

Obesity is often thought to have a negative impact on self-esteem because of the associated social stigmatization in western society. Constant comparison with an unrealistic societal ideal is assumed to negatively influence an obese individual's feelings of self-worth. However, studies examining the self-esteem of obese individuals have produced mixed results.

In adults, studies have generally failed to show significant differences between the self-esteem of obese and non-obese groups (Friedman and Brownell, 1995; Sarwer, Wadden and Foster, 1998). The number of studies that have investigated self-esteem in obese adults is small, however, and the majority are limited by methodological problems such as the use of a variety of (often unstandardized) measures of self-esteem, small sample sizes and a failure to examine gender differences or to take other confounding variables into account.

In children, studies of the effect of obesity on self-esteem are also inconclusive. French, Story and Perry (1995) reviewed 35 studies on self-esteem and obesity in children and adolescents, and found no clear and consistent outcome. Fewer than half of the studies reviewed showed significantly lower self-esteem in obese children and adolescents, with the clearest effects occurring in adolescents. Once again, these inconclusive results may be the result of methodological limitations. For example, many of the studies reviewed had relatively small sample sizes, and the definition of overweight varied enormously. In addition, the measures of self-esteem used in most of these studies are problematic. Most established measures of self-esteem aggregate responses to yield a single global score. This is based on the assumption that self-esteem is a global construct, rather than a multidimensional construct that takes into account self-evaluation in several different life domains (e.g. physical appearance self-esteem and academic competence self-esteem). The majority of the studies reviewed by French, Story and Perry (1995) assessed global rather than domain-specific self-esteem so they may have lacked the specificity to detect impairment of the specific aspects of self-esteem that are most closely related to obesity. Only a very small number of studies have used a multidimensional measure of self-esteem, such as the Harter Self-Perception Profile for Children (SPPC), to assess aspects of self-esteem in obese children. These studies have all found that physical appearance self-esteem (and in some cases athletic competence self-esteem), but not global self-esteem, was affected by being overweight (Hill, Draper and Stack, 1994).

By adolescence, however, this profile of reduced physical appearance self-esteem but preserved global self-esteem appears to have changed. In a longitudinal survey of over 1,500 children, Strauss (2000) found that, although there were no differences in global self-esteem between obese and non-obese 9- to 10-year-old children, by age 13–14 years obese children (both boys and girls) showed significantly decreased levels of global self-esteem compared with their non-obese counterparts. Using the SPPC, French *et al.* (1996) found that a higher BMI in teenage girls was not only associated with reduced self-esteem in the domains of physical appearance, athletic competence and romantic appeal, but was also associated with lower global self-esteem. This observation may suggest a developmental lag in the effects of obesity on global self-esteem relative to physical appearance self-esteem. It may be that self-evaluations of physical appearance become inextricably linked to global self-esteem from adolescence onwards.

Binge eating and other eating disorder symptoms

A third problem that is thought to occur with increased frequency among obese people is binge eating, defined as the frequent and regular intake of an objectively large amount of food with an associated sense of loss of control over eating. Indeed, it seems that one of the main adverse psychological consequences of childhood obesity may be the increased risk of eating disorder symptoms, particularly among girls (Friedman and Brownell, 1995). However, the links between eating disorders and childhood obesity need to be clarified. Childhood obesity has been identified as a significant risk factor for the development of eating disorders such as bulimia nervosa and binge eating disorder (BED) (Fairburn *et al.*, 1997, 1998), and a substantial number of obese adults with BED report the onset of strict dieting, binge eating or both during childhood, prior to the onset of their problems with obesity (Fairburn *et al.*, 1998). Prospective studies are needed to clarify the onset and course of binge eating and other eating-related problems in overweight/obese children.

Binge eating appears to be a relatively common problem among both male and female adolescents seeking treatment for obesity; however, there are large discrepancies in the prevalence rates reported, which are most likely attributable to differing definitions of binge eating and the variety of assessment instruments used. Estimates of the prevalence of binge eating among adolescents attending treatment for obesity range from 18–35 per cent for males and 27–57 per cent for females (Berkowitz, Stunkard and Stallings, 1993).

Relatively few studies have investigated the prevalence of binge eating in obese children under 13 years. Decaluwé, Braet and Fairburn (2003) found that 37 per cent of children (10–16 years) seeking treatment for their obesity reported binge eating, with 6 per cent reporting two or more episodes a week. This study, however, used self-report to assess binge eating behaviour, and the accuracy of self-reports of binge eating is uncertain, particularly in children. Research using a structured face-to-face clinical interview reported a much lower rate of 9 per cent (Decaluwé and Braet, 2003).

Research suggests that overweight and obese children who report binge eating have a higher rate of psychopathology than those who report no binge eating, including increased depression, anxiety, difficulties in social relationships, lower self-esteem, and greater eating, weight, and shape concerns (Berkowitz, Stunkard and Stallings, 1993; Decaluwé and Braet, 2003; Decaluwé, Braet and Fairburn, 2003). Whereas some studies have found that obese children who binge eat are significantly heavier than those who do not (Decaluwé and Braet, 2003), others have found no relationship between binge eating status and degree of overweight (Decaluwé, Braet and Fairburn, 2003). Research is needed to clarify the extent to which binge eaters are a distinctive subgroup of overweight and obese children and adolescents.

There are two main theories relating to the development and maintenance of binge eating: restraint theory and affect regulation theory. Restraint theory suggests that strict dietary restraint (dieting) and the adoption of rigid and inflexible dietary rules predispose people to binge eat for both physiological and psychological reasons. There is ample evidence that this pathway is a critical one in the aetiology of binge eating. Affect regulation theory suggests that some individuals binge eat in order to regulate negative affect such as sadness, anger or anxiety, or to distract themselves from unpleasant thoughts or emotions. Rather than acknowledging mood changes and suitably dealing with them, these individuals attempt to regulate their affect by eating. In lay terms this is often referred to as 'comfort eating'. It is also possible that the combination of dietary restraint and the tendency to use food to regulate negative affect may result in an increased vulnerability to binge eating.

The roles that dietary restraint and affect regulation play in binge eating in obese children and adolescents are unclear. In a two-year prospective study of risk factors for binge eating in adolescent girls, Stice, Presnell and Spangler (2002) found that strict dieting predicted the onset of binge eating. On the other hand, other studies of treatment-seeking obese children and adolescents have found no differences in the dieting histories of those who engage in binge eating and those who do not (Berkowitz, Stunkard and Stallings, 1993; Decaluwé, Braet and Fairburn, 2003). To our knowledge, no published study has explored whether some children binge eat in an attempt to regulate their affect.

Conclusions

It is now acknowledged that social and psychological problems may be the most common and damaging forms of morbidity associated with childhood obesity. In addition it seems that many of the psychosocial consequences of obesity are apparent even prior to adolescence. These adverse consequences include discrimination, exposure to teasing, peer relationship difficulties, low self-esteem, body dissatisfaction and the presence of binge eating. Further research is needed to investigate the extent, nature and severity of psychosocial problems that are associated with obesity in children. It is critical that we include these psychosocial needs, along with weight management, as a legitimate treatment goal for obese children.

Little research has attempted to identify the ways in which psychosocial factors may interact with a range of biological, behavioural and environmental factors to form causal pathways to the development and persistence of childhood obesity. A small number of previous studies have been able to suggest some psychosocial factors that may contribute to the development of obesity, such as low socioeconomic status, poor quality housing, a familial environment marked by neglectfulness, parental attitudes toward weight, shape and dieting, and parental control over a child's dietary intake. There is a need for carefully designed prospective studies to identify and test the whole range of psychosocial factors that may influence the development and persistence of obesity. These factors may include the presence of binge eating and other eating disorder symptoms, low self-esteem, unrealistic weight goals, over-evaluation of shape and weight, and intolerance of negative mood states. Future research will hopefully shed more light on the role that these potentially important risk factors play in the development and persistence of obesity.

References

Berkowitz, R., Stunkard, A.J. and Stallings, V.A. (1993) 'Binge eating disorder in obese adolescent girls', *Annals of the New York Academy of Sciences*, 699: 200–6.

Booth, M.L., Macaskill, P., Lazarus, R. and Baur, L.A. (1999) 'Sociodemographic distribution of measures of body fatness among children and adolescents in New South Wales, Australia', *International Journal of Obesity and Related Metabolic Disorders*, 23: 456–62.

Bruch, H. (1973) *Eating Disorders, Obesity, Anorexia Nervosa and the Person Within*, New York: Basic Books.

Carpenter, K.M., Hasin, D.S., Allison, D.B. and Faith, M.S. (2000) 'Relationships between obesity and DSM-IV major depressive disorder, suicide ideation and suicide attempts: results from a general population study', *American Journal of Public Health*, 90: 251–7.

Constanzo, P.R. and Woody, E.Z. (1985) 'Domain-specific parenting styles and their impact on the child's development of particular deviance: the example of obesity proneness', *Journal of Social and Clinical Psychology*, 3: 425–45.

Decaluwé, V. and Braet, C. (2003) 'Prevalence of binge-eating disorder in obese children and adolescents seeking weight-loss treatment', *International Journal of Obesity*, 27: 404–9.

Decaluwé, V., Braet, C. and Fairburn, C.G. (2003) 'Binge eating in obese children and adolescents', *International Journal of Eating Disorders*, 33: 78–84.

Fairburn, C.G., Welch, S.L., Doll, H.A., Davies, B.A. and O'Connor, M.E. (1997) 'Risk factors for bulimia nervosa: a community-based case-control study', *Archives of General Psychiatry*, 54: 509–17.

Fairburn, C.G., Doll, H.A., Welch, S.L., Hay, P.J., Davies, B.A. and O'Connor, M.E. (1998) 'Risk factors for binge eating disorder: a community-based case-control study', *Archives of General Psychiatry*, 55: 425–32.

French, S.A., Story, M. and Perry, C.L. (1995) 'Self-esteem and obesity in children and adolescents: a literature review', *Obesity Research*, 3: 479–90.

French, S.A., Perry, C.L., Leon, G.R. and Fulkerson, J.A. (1996) 'Self-esteem and changes in body mass index over three years in a cohort of adolescents', *Obesity Research*, 4: 27–33.

Friedman, M.A. and Brownell, K.D. (1995) 'Psychological correlates of obesity: moving to the next generation', *Psychological Bulletin*, 117: 3–20.

Gortmaker, S.L., Must, A., Perrin, J.M., Sobal, A.M. and Dietz, W.H. (1993) 'Social and economic consequences of overweight in adolescence and young adulthood', *New England Journal of Medicine*, 329: 1008–12.

Grilo, C.M., Wilfley, D.E., Brownell, K.D. and Rodin, J. (1994) 'Teasing, body image, and self-esteem in a clinical sample of obese women', *Addictive Behaviours*, 19: 443–50.

Hill, A.J. and Pallin, V. (1998) 'Dieting awareness and low self-worth: related issues in 8-year-old girls', *International Journal of Eating Disorders*, 24: 405–13.

Hill, A.J., Draper, E. and Stack, J. (1994) 'A weight on children's minds: body shape dissatisfaction at 9 years-old', *International Journal of Obesity*, 18: 383–9.

Hill, A.J. and Silver, E. (1995) 'Fat, friendless and unhealthy: 9-year-old children's perception of body shape stereotypes', *International Journal of Obesity*, 19: 423–30.

Johnson, S.L. and Birch, L.L. (1994) 'Parents' and children's adiposity and eating style', *Pediatrics*, 94: 653–61.

Lissau, I. and Sorenson, T.I.A. (1994) 'Parental neglect during childhood and increased risk of obesity in young adulthood', *Lancet*, 343: 324–7.

Mendelson, B.K., White, D.R. and Schliecker, E. (1995) 'Adolescents' weight, sex, and family functioning', *International Journal of Eating Disorders*, 17: 73–9.

Mustillo, S., Worthman, C., Erkanli, A., Keeler, G., Angold, A. and Costello, J. (2003) 'Obesity and psychiatric disorder: developmental trajectories', *Pediatrics*, 111: 851–9.

Pike, K.M. and Rodin, J. (1991) 'Mothers, daughters and disordered eating', *Journal of Abnormal Psychology*, 100: 198–204.

Richardson, S.A., Goodman, N., Hastorf, A.H. and Dornbusch, S.M. (1961) 'Cultural uniformity in reaction to physical disabilities', *American Sociological Review*, 26: 241–7.

Sarwer, D.B., Wadden, T.A. and Foster, G.D. (1998) 'Assessment of body image dissatisfaction in obese women: specificity, severity, and clinical significance', *Journal of Consulting and Clinical Psychology*, 66: 651–4.

Sobal, J. and Stunkard, A.J. (1989) 'Socioeconomic status and obesity: a review of the literature', *Psychological Bulletin*, 105: 260–75.

Stafferi, J.R. (1967) 'A study of social stereotype of body image in children', *Journal of Personality and Social Psychology*, 7: 101–4.

Stice, E., Presnell, K. and Spangler, D. (2002) 'Risk factors for binge eating onset in adolescent girls: a 2-year prospective investigation', *Health Psychology*, 21: 131–8.

Stice, E., Cameron, R.P., Hayward, C., Barr-Taylor, C. and Killen, J.D. (1999) 'Naturalistic weight-reduction efforts prospectively predict growth in relative weight and onset of obesity among female adolescents', *Journal of Consulting and Clinical Psychology*, 67: 967–74.

Strauss, R.S. (2000) 'Childhood obesity and self-esteem', *Pediatrics*, 105: 15.

Wilfley, D.M., Stein, R.I., Hayden, H.A., Douchnis, J.Z. and Zabinski, M.F. (1998) 'Social consequences of childhood obesity', *International Journal of Obesity*, 22(Suppl 4): S15.

8 Physical activity, appetite control and energy balance

Implications for obesity

N.A. King

Introduction

As was the case over 50 years ago (Kennedy, 1953), issues associated with energy balance (EB) regulation, homeostasis and implications for obesity continue to attract interest (Macias, 2004). Homeostasis is based on the concept that body weight has a 'set-point' and that, following any perturbations in EB, body weight will return to baseline. The work of Edholm and Mayer in the 1950s contributed significantly to the understanding of EB and body weight regulation (Edholm 1957; Edholm et al., 1954; Mayer et al., 1954, 1956). In particular, Edholm demonstrated that there were marked variations in daily energy intake (EI) and energy expenditure (EE) suggesting that acute (i.e. day-to-day) EB is not tightly regulated (Edholm et al., 1970). Despite this acute uncoupling, there tends to be synchrony between EE and EI, and hence body weight, over a slightly longer time period (e.g. a week). Therefore, there is some indication that body weight is regulated. Counter to this is the current obesity epidemic and increase in prevalence of childhood obesity (Hedley et al., 2004), which implies that body weight is not tightly regulated, or at least not in some susceptible individuals.

Physical activity and energy balance regulation

In light of the obesity problem, there is a focus on public health messages and recommendations in an attempt to increase physical activity levels. Therefore, the effect of increased physical activity on appetite sensitivity and energy balance regulation is an important consideration. Increases or decreases in activity EE will automatically create an acute perturbation to the EB system. It is the detection of and compensation for these changes that define the sensitivity of the EB regulatory system. Inter-individual variability in the ability of the regulatory system to compensate for perturbations in EB could partly explain why, for some individuals, exercise often produces disappointing effects on body weight.

Appetite sensitivity is how precise the appetite system is in detecting when the body has consumed enough energy. It is possible that habitually physically active individuals are better able to regulate their food intake and energy balance because of increased appetite sensitivity. Mayer, Roy and Mitra (1956) were the first to highlight the flaw in the belief that EI functions in such a way that it automatically increases following an increase in EE and decreases following a reduction in EE. In their study of jute mill workers in West Bengal, Mayer, Roy and Mitra (1956) found that EI increases with activity only within a certain zone of activity ('normal activity'), and that below this range ('sedentary zone') a decrease in activity is not associated with a decrease in EI. Rather, it is associated with an increase in EI combined with an increase in body weight.

More recently, Long, Hart and Morgan (2002) demonstrated that habitually physically active individuals have an increased accuracy of short-term regulation of EI in comparison to inactive individuals. In this study, participants were given either a low- or high-energy preload for lunch, and were then asked to eat *ad libitum* from a test meal buffet. EI from the buffet did not significantly differ following the two preloads in the non-exercise group, showing a negligible compensation (approximately 7 per cent). On the other hand, the habitually active group reduced their EI following the high-energy preload compared to the low-energy preload, exhibiting approximately 90 per cent compensation. This suggests that regular physical activity may increase sensitivity to satiety signals, and that EI is more tightly regulated. Therefore, being physically active could have positive implications for improving the regulation of EB, independent of the associated increase in EE.

Physical activity and obesity

A physically active lifestyle, whether as a child or adolescent, is conducive to a healthy lifestyle and preventing disease (Chakravarthy and Booth, 2004), whereas a sedentary lifestyle is associated with chronic disease and ill health (Twisk, 2001). There is currently a paradox that, despite growing health concerns and an increase in the publicity of physical activity recommendations, a majority of Australians remain physically inactive (Armstrong, Bauman and Davies, 2000). Indeed, there is a trend towards an increase in sedentary, inactive lifestyles across most of the developed countries (AIHW, 2004). Unfortunately, the opportunity for many youngsters to be physically active has reduced over time, probably as a result of a series of changing environmental factors. Previous research has found that the environment exerts a strong influence on physical activity (Dollman, Norton and Norton, 2005). In particular, children are at risk from their susceptibility to a technologically changing environment that facilitates an inactive lifestyle. For example, in Australian children, active transport levels are very low (Harten and Olds, 2004). In addition, the EE associated with incidental activity is decreasing in children on account of the widespread use of labour-saving devices, playing computer games and watching television (ABS, 2001). Physical activity and food are basic necessities for survival; however, cultural changes in many parts of the world have 'engineered' spontaneous physical activity out of the daily lives of many (Chakravarthy and Booth, 2004). The indication is that, collectively, behaviours undertaken by children are predominantly sedentary in nature and involve minimal

EE. A combination of environmental pressures, technological factors and societal transitions from childhood to adolescence are likely to promote sedentary behaviour that could potentially lead to weight gain (Jebb and Moore, 1999).

Despite the speculation and anecdotal evidence, there is a lack of comparable and robust data to demonstrate that the actual level of physical activity (and EE) in today's children is low compared with their counterparts several decades ago. This is an area which has attracted some controversy, mainly because of the lack of a 'benchmark' of physical activity with which to compare current levels (Ekelund, Brage and Wareham, 2004; Wilkin and Voss, 2004). Most of the evidence comes from indirect surrogate measures (Prentice and Jebb, 1995). For example, walking and cycling to school are replaced by car transportation (DETR, 2000; Harten and Olds, 2004). However, there is some direct evidence that, like adults, many children do not participate in appropriate levels of physical activity (Jackson et al., 2002; Montgomery et al., 2002; Pratt, Macera and Blanton, 1999; Reilly and McDowell, 2003; Reilly et al., 2004) and that activity levels are lower than recommendations (Salbe et al., 1997). The indications are that, for today's children, physical activity levels are low and, more importantly, progressively decreasing. If this trend occurs in synergy with an increase in EI, levels of overweight and obesity will escalate (Hills, 1995; Pařízková and Hills, 2001, 2005). Efforts should be concentrated on facilitating an active lifestyle for children in an attempt to put a stop to the increasing prevalence of obese children (Graf et al., 2004). Health strategies and initiatives are required to reduce sedentary behaviours, a reduction which in theory should automatically increase activity (Epstein and Roemmich, 2001).

Because of methodological problems associated with the validity and accuracy of measuring physical activity per se, it is difficult to prove a direct link between a sedentary lifestyle and weight gain. Thus, the evidence for a causal link between 'sedentariness' and obesity in adults is weak (Fogelholm and Kukkonen-Harjula, 2000; Parsons et al., 1999). However, there is some evidence that sedentary behaviours are associated with overweight and obesity in children (Livingstone et al., 2003; Strong et al., 2005). For example, TV viewing is associated with lower habitual physical activity and cardiorespiratory fitness (Dietz and Gortmaker, 1985; Gortmaker et al., 1996) and increased obesity (Kimm et al., 2005; Moore et al., 2003). In contrast, it has been suggested that sedentary and active behaviours can coexist (Biddle et al., 2004); and that one type (i.e. sedentary or active) of behaviour does not automatically displace the other. For example, it is possible for children to combine physically active behaviours (e.g. participation in sport and exercise) with sedentary behaviours (e.g. computer games, watching television) within the same day. Consequently, there is some controversy over the true, direct effect of sedentary behaviours on weight gain and obesity in children (Biddle et al., 2004).

Despite a lack of concrete and robust evidence to prove a causal association, it is intuitive that sedentary behaviours in children should be limited because of their contribution to a reduction in EE and promotion of a positive energy balance. One of the key features of sedentary behaviours is that they typically coexist with eating, which in turn could augment the obesity epidemic (Blundell, King and Bryant, 2005). Recent evidence supports this phenomenon by demonstrating that sedentary behaviours are associated with a higher snack intake in children and adolescents (Rennie and Jebb, 2003). Reduced activity and concomitant poor food choice are contributing to an increase in overweight and obesity, particularly in the developed world. A recent phenomenon in developing countries is the combination of underweight children and overweight adults, frequently coexisting in the same family (Caballero, 2004).

Physical activity and appetite control

It is commonly assumed that physical activity is an ineffective strategy for losing weight since the energy expended will drive up hunger and food intake to compensate for the energy deficit incurred. In this regard, the compensatory increase in EI is assumed to be the main cause of a lack of weight loss. It is logical to infer that, by creating an energy deficit, physical activity will have a similar effect on EB as a dietary-induced energy deficit. There are many examples in the literature of dietary-induced reductions in EI giving rise to compensatory increases in hunger and food intake (Delargy et al., 1995; Green, Burley and Blundell, 1994; Hubert, King and Blundell, 1998).

There are several ways in which exercise could potentially cause changes in EI. These include increased frequency of eating (e.g. snacking), increased portion size and increased energy density of food. Exercise could also alter macronutrient preferences and food choices. This might be expected as a drive to seek particular foods to replenish short-term energy stores, and could be reflected in the macronutrient composition of the diet selected following episodes of physical activity (King and Blundell, 1995; Tremblay et al., 1989).

Contrary to belief, there is no immediate compensatory increase in hunger and EI response to an exercise-induced energy deficit (Imbeault et al., 1997; King, Burley and Blundell, 1994; King and Blundell, 1995; King et al., 1996, 1997; Kissileff et al., 1990; Lluch, King and Blundell, 1998; Reger, Allison and Kurucz, 1984; Thompson, Wolfe and Eikelboom, 1988; Westerterp-Plantenga et al., 1997). This phenomenon is not limited to adults. Acute impositions in exercise also failed to create an increase in EI in 9- to 10-year-olds (Moore et al., 2002). Therefore, the overall body of evidence points to a loose coupling between exercise-induced EE and EI (Blundell and King, 1998; Blundell et al., 2003; King, Tremblay and Blundell, 1997; King, 1998).

Two criticisms of these short-term studies are that they fail to track EI for a sufficiently long period following the increased physical activity interventions, and that the exercise-induced increase in EE is not large enough to stimulate appetite. However, even with a high dose of exercise (gross exercise-induced increase in EE of 4.6 MJ) in a single day and tracking EI for the following two days, there is no automatic compensatory rise in hunger and EI (King et al., 1997). Therefore, the evidence that an acute exercise-induced negative EB is not compensated for by an increase in EI is relatively robust. One reason for this loose coupling is that the behavioural act of eating is held in place by environmental contingencies and short-term post-ingestive physiological responses arising from eating itself. In support of this is the tendency for eating and activity behaviours to return to their original habitual level following interventions which intentionally create a negative energy balance (Speakman, Stubbs and Mercer, 2002).

Although overall the evidence from the acute studies indicates that EI is not immediately driven up by increased physical activity, a series of seminal papers by Stubbs *et al.* demonstrated that partial compensation starts to occur if physical activity persists for long enough. The evidence confirmed that over a period of seven days (Stubbs *et al.*, 2002a,b) and 14 days (Stubbs *et al.*, 2004a), EI did not remain constant following the marked elevation of EE. Findings from the 14-day exercise intervention suggested that, on average, subjects compensated for ≈30 per cent of the exercise-induced energy deficit (Stubbs *et al.*, 2004a). However, there was considerable variation in the extent of compensation between individuals such that some compensated completely (100 per cent) for the increase in EE. More recently, a combination of increased activity and restricted diet for six weeks caused a significant increase in hunger in obese children attending a residential obesity camp (King, Hester and Gately, 2007). Thus, although most of the evidence from acute studies indicates that physical activity interventions fail to drive up hunger and EI, there is emerging evidence to indicate that they are sensitive to longer-term imposed energy deficits.

The loose coupling between exercise-induced EE and EI has positive implications for weight control for increases in EE. Unfortunately, it has negative implications for decreases in EE. When EE automatically decreases in individuals who become sedentary, EI is not down-regulated to a new lower level in equilibrium with the reduced EE. Experimentally induced, imposed reductions in EE can be simulated when individuals reside in a whole body calorimeter. A short-term study (Murgatroyd *et al.*, 1999) and a medium-term study (Stubbs *et al.*, 2004b) have demonstrated that activity-induced reductions in EE are not compensated for by a concomitant reduction in EI. Therefore, physical inactivity does not automatically reduce food intake. The implications for weight gain and obesity are of particular concern, especially in light of the evidence that inactivity-induced reductions in EE are occurring naturally in the free-living environment because people are becoming less active. Considering that eating tends to be a sedentary activity, inactivity could even increase EI; especially energy-dense snack foods (Rennie and Jebb, 2003). Thus, sedentariness could be a risk factor for two reasons: a natural decrease in EE and an increase in EI due to consumption of energy-dense foods.

The role of physical activity in weight control

The weak coupling between activity-induced EE and EI generates an optimistic view of the role of exercise in weight control and preventing weight gain. Therefore, from a practical perspective, physical activity should be a successful method of weight loss. However, physical activity often produces disappointing effects on body weight. There may be a number of reasons why this is the case. For example, a failure to maintain a 100 per cent compliance with the exercise regime, and a reduction in physical activity in the non-exercise time (recovery periods) could both contribute to a lack of weight loss. Inappropriate food choices and allowance of food rewards, as well as misjudgments about the rate of eating-induced intake (calories consumed) relative to the energy cost of physical activity (calories expended) could also jeopardize the outcome. Some individuals make poor evaluations of the amount of energy that can be expended during exercise, and the amount that can be ingested during eating. For a fixed level of energy the duration of exercise (expenditure) is markedly greater compared with the duration of eating (intake). For example, to expend 600 kcal, an individual of moderate fitness (i.e. VO_2max 3 L/min) would have to exercise for approximately 60 minutes at 75 per cent VO_2max. However, any individual (independent of aerobic fitness) could ingest 600 kcal of food energy in the form of an energy-dense snack (e.g. a Danish pastry or a couple of doughnuts) in three to four minutes. Consequently, individuals should be informed about the possible 'mismatch' between the rate of EE (low) and rate of EI (high).

Food choice must be controlled independently of increasing physical activity; an increase in physical activity does not automatically protect against inappropriate food choice. Several studies have demonstrated that the beneficial effects of exercise on energy balance can be completely reversed when physical activity is combined with high-fat, energy-dense foods and diets (King, Burley and Blundell, 1994; Murgatroyd *et al.*, 1999; Tremblay *et al.*, 1994). An increase in physical activity does not automatically protect against inappropriate food choice. Therefore, physical activity should not be viewed as an opportunity to abandon any restraint over eating, nor to indulge excessively on available foods.

It is unlikely that activity-induced appetite responses will be identical in all individuals. Inter-individual variability is likely to render people either resistant or susceptible to the weight control-related benefits of exercise. Most studies evaluating the efficacy of exercise on weight loss report the mean data only and inadvertently fail to identify the inter-individual variability. Very few studies express the data individually, or at least further explore the data in search of sub-groups or individual variability. Using body weight as a marker of success, previous studies have identified good 'responders' and 'maintainers' (Snyder *et al.*, 1997; Weinsier *et al.*, 2002). EI has also been used as a marker of regulation (compensators and non-compensators) in response to exercise (Stubbs *et al.*, 2004a). Therefore, it is important to examine the individual responses to exercise interventions.

Conclusion

There is no doubt that a physically active lifestyle, whether as a child or an adolescent, contributes to a healthy lifestyle and prevents disease (Chakravarthy and Booth, 2004). The association between inactivity and weight gain is less clear; however, this should not undermine the importance of promoting physical activity on account of its important role in the prevention of weight gain. There is strong evidence for a loose coupling between activity-induced EE and EI. This has optimistic implications for the use of exercise in weight control, but is a problem for a nation that is becoming increasingly sedentary. This latter implication strengthens the need for strategies to increase physical activity and to reduce sedentary behaviours. Importantly, physical activity has the potential to be a successful method of obesity prevention, but only if there is compliance with the prescribed amount, together with judicious control over food choice that involves selection of low- to medium-energy-dense diets.

However, the message should be accompanied by a warning that the delivery of the message does not ensure its implementation. Initially, there must be a realistic appreciation of the energy cost associated with physical activity and exercise compared with the energy content of food consumed. The widespread overestimation of the amount of energy used up by exercise, coupled with the underestimation of the amount of energy consumed in foods, generates a misleading impression of the amount of behavioural control required for energy balance and weight control. Secondly, it should be recognized that some individuals have the capacity to benefit from exercise more than others. Some individuals will be more resistant to physical activity interventions and will need additional or alternative strategies to help them reach a target of a more healthy weight. There needs to be a much greater understanding of individual human variability (in children and in adults) before the appropriate health messages can be effective.

References

ABS (Australian Bureau of Statistics) (2001) *Children's Participation in Cultural and Leisure Activities, Australia*, cat. no. 4901.0, Canberra: ABS.

AIHW (Australian Institute of Health and Welfare) (2004) *A Rising Epidemic: Overweight and Obesity in Australian Children and Adolescents*, Risk Factors Data Briefing 2, Canberra: AIHW.

Armstrong, T., Bauman A. and Davies, J. (2000) *Physical Activity Patterns of Australian Adults. Results of the 1999 National Physical Activity Survey*, Canberra: Australian Institute of Health and Welfare.

Biddle, S.J., Gorely, T., Marshall, S.J., Murdey, I. and Cameron, N. (2004) 'Physical activity and sedentary behaviours in youth: issues and controversies', *Journal of the Royal Society for the Promotion of Health*, 124: 29–33.

Blundell, J.E. and King, N.A. (1998) 'Effects of exercise on appetite control: loose coupling between energy expenditure and energy intake', *International Journal of Obesity*, 22: 1–8.

Blundell, J.E., King, N.A. and Bryant, E. (2005) 'Interactions among physical activity food choice and appetite control: health message in physical activity and diet', in N. Caero, N.G. Norgan, G.T.H. Ellison (eds) *Childhood Obesity*, London: Taylor & Francis, pp. 135–48.

Blundell, J.E., Stubbs, R.J, Hughes, D.A., Whybrow, S. and King, N.A. (2003) 'Cross talk between physical activity and appetite control: does physical activity stimulate appetite?', *Proceedings of the Nutrition Society*, 62: 651–61.

Caballero, B. (2004) 'A nutrition paradox – undernutrition and obesity in developing countries', *New England Journal of Medicine*, 352: 1514–16.

Chakravarthy, M.V. and Booth, F.W. (2004) 'Eating, exercise, and "thrifty" genotypes: connecting the dots toward an evolutionary understanding of modern chronic diseases', *Journal of Applied Physiology*, 96: 3–10.

Delargy, H.D., Burley, V.J., Sullivan, K.R., Fletcher, R.J. and Blundell, JE. (1995) 'Effects of different soluble : insoluble fibre ratios at breakfast on 24-h pattern of dietary intake and satiety', *European Journal of Clinical Nutrition*, 49: 754–66.

DETR (Department of the Environment, Transport and the Regions) (2000) *National Transport Survey: Update 1997/1999*, London: The Stationery Office.

Dietz, W.H. and Gortmaker, S.L. (1985) 'Do we fatten our children at the TV set? Obesity and television viewing in children and adolescents', *Pediatrics*, 75: 807–12.

Dollman, J., Norton, K. and Norton, L. (2005) 'Evidence for secular trends in children's physical activity behaviour', *British Journal of Sports Medicine*, 39: 892–7.

Edholm, O.G. (1957) 'Energy balance in man', *Journal of Human Nutrition*, 1: 413–31.

Edholm, O.G., Fletcher, J.G., Widdowson, E.M. and McCance, R.A. (1954) 'The energy expenditure and food intake of individual men', *British Journal of Nutrition*, 9: 286–300.

Edholm, O.G., Adam, J.M., Healy, M.J.R., Wolff, H.S. Goldsmith, R. and Best, T.W. (1970) 'Food intake and energy expenditure of army recruits', *British Journal of Nutrition*, 24: 1091–1107.

Ekelund, U., Brage, S. and Wareham, N.J. (2004) 'Physical activity in young children', *Lancet*, 363: 1162.

Epstein, L.H. and Roemmich, J.N. (2001) 'Reducing sedentary behaviour: role of modifying physical activity', *Exercise and Sports Science Reviews*, 29: 103–8.

Fogelholm, M. and Kukkonen-Harjula, K. (2000) 'Does physical activity prevent weight gain? A systematic review', *Obesity Research*, 1: 95–111.

Gortmaker, S.L., Must, A., Sobol, A.M., Peterson, K., Colditz, G.A. and Dietz, W.H. (1996) 'Television viewing as a cause of increasing obesity among children in the United States', *Archives of Pediatric and Adolescent Medicine*, 150: 356–62.

Graf, C., Koch, B., Kretschmann-Kandel, E., Falkowski, G., Christ, H., Coburger, S., Lehmacher, W., Bjarnason-Wehrens, B., Platen, P., Tokarski, W., Predel, H.G. and Dordel, S (2004) 'Correlation between BMI, leisure habits and motor abilities in childhood (CHILT-Project)', *International Journal of Obesity*, 28: 22–6.

Green, S.M., Burley, S.M. and Blundell, J.E. (1994) 'Effect of fat and sucrose-containing foods on the size of eating episodes and energy intake in lean males: potential for causing overconsumption', *European Journal of Clinical Nutrition*, 48: 547–55.

Harten, N. and Olds, T. (2004) 'Patterns of active transport in 11–12 year old Australian children', *Australian and New Zealand Journal of Public Health*, 28: 167–72.

Hedley, A.A., Ogden, C.L., Johnson, C.L., Carroll, M.D., Curtin, L.R. and Flegal, K.M. (2004) 'Prevalence of overweight and obesity among US children, adolescents, and adults, 1999–2002', *Journal of American Medical Association*, 291: 2847–50.

Hills, A.P (1995) 'Education for preventing obesity', *Journal of International Council for Health, Physical Education, Recreation, Sport and Dance*, 30: 30–2.

Hubert, P., King, N.A. and Blundell, J.E. (1998) 'Uncoupling the effects of energy expenditure and energy intake: appetite response to short-term energy deficit induced by meal omission and physical activity', *Appetite*, 31: 9–19.

Imbeault, P., Saint-Pierre, S., Almeras, N., Tremblay, A. (1997) 'Acute effects of exercise on energy intake and feeding behaviour', *British Journal of Nutrition*, 77: 511–21.

Jackson, D.M., Reilly, J.J., Kelly, L.A., Montgomery, C., Grant, S. and Paton, J.Y. (2002) 'Objectively measured habitual physical activity and inactivity in a representative sample of 3–4 year old children', *Proceedings of the Nutrition Society*, 61: 154A.

Jebb, S.A. and Moore, M.S. (1999) 'Contribution of a sedentary lifestyle and inactivity to the etiology of overweight and obesity: current evidence and research issue', *Medicine and Science in Sports Exercise*, 31: S534–41.

Kennedy, G.C. (1953) 'The role of depot fat in the hypothalamic control of food intake in the rat', *Proceedings of the Royal Society of London*, 140B: 578–92.

Kimm, S.Y.S., Glynn, N.W., Obarzanek, E., Kriska, A.M., Daniels, S.R., Barton, B.A. and Liu, K. (2005) 'Relationship between the changes in physical activity and body-mass index during adolescence: a multicentre longitudinal study', *Lancet*, 366: 301–7.

King, N.A. (1998) 'The relationship between physical activity and food intake', *Proceedings of the Nutrition Society*, 57: 1–9.

King, N.A. and Blundell, J.E. (1995) 'High-fat foods overcome the energy expenditure due to exercise after cycling and running', *European Journal of Clinical Nutrition*, 49: 114–23.

King, N.A., Burley, V.J. and Blundell, J.E. (1994) 'Exercise-induced suppression of appetite: effects on food intake and implications for energy balance', *European Journal of Clinical Nutrition*, 48: 715–24.

King, N.A., Hester, J. and Gately, P.J. (2007) 'The effect of a medium term activity- and diet-induced energy deficit on subjective appetite sensations in obese children', *International Journal of Obesity and Related Metabolic Disorders*, 31: 334–9.

King, N.A., Tremblay, A. and Blundell, J.E. (1997) 'Effects of exercise on appetite control: implications for energy balance', *Medicine and Science in Sports and Exercise*, 29: 1076–89.

King, N.A., Snell, L., Smith, R.D. and Blundell, J.E. (1996) 'Effects of short-term exercise on appetite response in unrestrained females', *European Journal of Clinical Nutrition*, 50: 663–7.

King, N.A., Lluch, A. Stubbs, R.J. and Blundell, J.E. (1997) 'High dose exercise does not increase hunger or energy intake in free living males', *European Journal of Clinical Nutrition*, 51: 478–83.

Kissileff, H.R., Pi-Sunyer, X.F., Segal, K., Meltzer, S. and Foelsch, P.A. (1990) 'Acute effects of exercise on food intake in obese and non-obese women', *American Journal of Clinical Nutitrition*, 52: 240–5.

Livingstone, M.B., Robson, P.J., Wallace, J.M. and McKinley, M.C. (2003) 'How active are we? Levels of routine physical activity in children and adults', *Proceedings of the Nutrition Society*, 62: 681–701.

Lluch, A., King, N.A. and Blundell, J.E. (1998) 'Exercise in dietary restrained women: no effect on energy intake but change in hedonic ratings', *European Journal of Clinical Nutrition*, 52: 300–7.

Long, S.J., Hart, K. and Morgan, L.M. (2002) 'The ability of habitual exercisers to influence appetite and food intake in response to high- and low-energy preloads in man', *British Journal of Nutrition*, 87: 517–23.

Macias, A.E. (2004) 'Experimental demonstration of human weight homeostasis: implications for understanding obesity', *British Journal of Nutrition*, 91: 479–84.

Mayer, J., Roy, P. and Mitra, K.P. (1956) 'Relation between caloric intake, body weight, and physical work: studies in an industrial male population in West Bengal', *American Journal of Clinical Nutrition*, 4: 169–74.

Mayer, J., Marshall, N.B., Vitale, J.J., Christensen, J.H. Mashayekhi, M.B. and Stare, F.J. (1954) 'Exercise, food intake and body weight in normal and genetically obese adult mice', *American Journal of Physiology*, 177: 544.

Montgomery, C., Kelly, L.A., Jackson, D.M., Reilly, J.J., Grant, S. and Paton, J.Y. (2002)

'Changes in total energy expenditure in a representative sample of young children: a cross-sectional and longitudinal analysis', *Proceedings of the Nutrition Society*, 61: 160A.

Moore, M.S., Dodd, C.D., Welsman, J.R. and Armstrong, N. (2002) 'Lack of short-term compensation for imposed exercise in 9–10 year-old girls', *Proceedings of the Nutrition Society*, 61: 156A.

Moore, L.L., Di Gao, A.S., Bradle, M.A.S., Cupples, L.A., Sundarajan-Ramamurti, P.H.A., Proctor, M.H., Hood, M.Y., Singer, M.R. and Ellison, R.C. (2003) 'Does early physical activity predict body fat change throughout childhood?', *Preventative Medicine*, 37: 10–17.

Murgatroyd, P.R., Goldberg, G.R., Leahy, F.E., Gilsenan, M.B. and Prentice, A.M. (1999) 'Effects of inactivity and diet composition on human energy balance', *International Journal of Obesity and Related Metabolic Disorders*, 23: 1269–75.

Parízková, J. and Hills, A.P. (2001) *Childhood Obesity: Prevention and Management*, Boca Raton, FL: CRC Press.

Parízková, J. and Hills, A.P. (2005) *Childhood Obesity: Prevention and Management*, 2nd edition, Boca Raton, FL: CRC Press.

Parsons, T.J., Power, C., Logan, S. and Summerbell, C.D. (1999) 'Childhood predictors of adult obesity: a systematic review', *International Journal of Obesity*, 33: S1–107.

Pratt, M., Macera, C.A. and Blanton, C. (1999) 'Levels of physical activity and inactivity in children and adults in the United States: current evidence and research issues', *Medicine and Science in Sports and Exercise*, 31(Suppl): S526–33.

Prentice, A.M. and Jebb, S.A. (1995) 'Obesity in Britain: gluttony or sloth?', *British Medical Journal*, 311: 437–9.

Reger, W.E., Allison, T.A. and Kurucz, R.L. (1984) 'Exercise, post-exercise metabolic rate and appetite', *Sport Health and Nutrition*, 2: 115–23.

Reilly, J.J. and McDowell, Z.C. (2003) 'Physical activity interventions in the prevention and treatment of paediatric obesity: systematic review and critical appraisal', *Proceedings of the Nutrition Society*, 62: 611–19.

Reilly, J.J., Jackson, D.M., Montgomery, C., Kelly, L.A., Slater, C., Grant, S. and Paton, J.Y. (2004) 'Total energy expenditure and physical activity in young Scottish children: mixed longitudinal study', *Lancet*, 363: 211–12.

Rennie, K.L., and Jebb, S.A. (2003) 'Sedentary lifestyles are associated with being overweight and consumption of savoury snacks in young people (4–18 years)', *Proceedings of the Nutrition Society*, 62: 83A.

Salbe, A.D., Fontvieille, A.M., Harper, I.T. and Ravussin, E. (1997) 'Low levels of physical activity in 5-year-old children', *Journal of Pediatrics*, 131: 423–9.

Snyder, K.A., Donnelly, J.E., Jabobsen, D.J., Hertner, G. and Jakicic, J.M. (1997) 'The effects of long-term, moderate intensity, intermittent exercise on aerobic capacity, body composition, blood lipids, insulin and glucose on overweight females', *International Journal of Obesity*, 21: 1180–9.

Speakman, J.R., Stubbs, R.J. and Mercer, J.G. (2002) 'Does body mass play a role in the regulation of food intake?', *Proceedings of the Nutrition Society*, 61: 471–87.

Strong, W.B., Malina, R.M., Blimkie, C.J.R., Daniels, S.R., Dishman, R.K., Gutin, B., Hergenroeder, A.C., Must, A., Nixon, P.A., Pivarnik, J.M., Rowland, T., Trost, S. and Trudeau, F. (2005) 'Evidence based physical activity for school-age youth', *Journal of Pediatrics*, 146: 732–7.

Stubbs, R. J., Sepp, A., Hughes, D.A, Johnstone, A.M., King, N.A., Horgan, G. and Blundell, J.E. (2002a) 'The effect of graded levels of exercise on energy intake and balance in free-living women', *International Journal of Obesity and Related Metabolic Disorders*, 26: 866–9.

Stubbs, R.J., Sepp, A., Hughes, D.A., Johnstone, A.M., Horgan, G.W., King N. and Blundell J. (2002b) 'The effect of graded levels of exercise on energy intake and balance in free-living men, consuming their normal diet', *European Journal of Clinical Nutrition*, 56: 129–40.

Stubbs, R.J., Hughes, D.A., Johnstone, A.M., Whybrow, S., Horgan, G.W., King, N. and Blundell, J. (2004a) 'Rate and extent of compensatory changes in energy intake and expenditure in response to altered exercise and diet composition in humans', *American Journal of Physiology – Regulatory, Integrative and Comparative Physiology*, 286: R350–8.

Stubbs, R.J., Hughes, D.A., Ritz, P., Johnstone, A.M., Horgan, G.W., King, N. and Blundell, J.E. (2004b) 'A decrease in physical activity affects appetite, energy and nutrient balance in lean men feeding ad libitum', *American Journal of Clinical Nutrition*, 79: 62–9.

Thompson, D.A., Wolfe, L.A. and Eikelboom, R. (1988) 'Acute effects of exercise intensity on appetite in young men', *Medicine and Science in Sports and Exercise*, 20: 222–7.

Tremblay, A., Plourde, G., Despres, J.P. and Bouchard, C. (1989) 'Impact of dietary fat content and fat oxidation on energy intake in humans', *American Journal of Clinical Nutrition*, 49: 799–805.

Tremblay, A., Almeras, N., Boer, J., Kranenbarg, E.K. and Despres, J.P. (1994) 'Diet composition and postexercise energy balance', *American Journal of Clinical Nutrition*, 59: 975–9.

Twisk, J.W.R. (2001) 'Physical activity guidelines for children and adolescents. A critical review', *Sports Medicine*, 31: 617–27.

Weinsier, R.L., Hunter, G.R., Desmond, R.A.. Byrne, N.M., Zuckerman, P.A. and Darnell, B.E. (2002) 'Free-living activity energy expenditure in women successful and unsuccessful at maintaining a normal body weight', *American Journal of Clinical Nutrition*, 75: 499–504.

Westerterp-Plantenga, M.S., Verwegen, C.R.T., Ijedema, M.J.W., Wijckmans, N.E.G. and Saris, W.H.M. (1997) 'Acute effects of exercise or sauna on appetite in obese and non-obese men', *Physiology and Behaviour*, 62: 1345–54.

Wilkin, T. and Voss, L.D. (2004) 'Physical activity in young children', *Lancet*, 363: 1162–3.

9 Eating behaviour in children and the measurement of food intake

*J. Bressan, A.P. Hills and
H.H.M. Hermsdorff*

Introduction

There is a growing emphasis by clinicians and researchers on the lifestyle behaviours of children because of the relationship of these behaviours to adulthood diseases such as obesity, cardiovascular disease and osteoporosis (Hoek *et al.*, 2004; Schoeller, 2003; Wilson and Lewis, 2004). Trends in the food consumption patterns of children should be considered in the design and implementation of population-based behaviour strategies for the promotion of health and prevention of chronic diseases beginning in childhood (Nicklas *et al.*, 2004). Well-established methods of food intake assessment need to be continually modified because of the rapidly changing patterns of food consumption and dietary composition within contemporary populations (Willett, 1998). An important component of such work is to study the relationship between diet and disease in epidemiological studies.

Diet is very complex and difficult to measure. Several methods have been developed to assess intake, but no method is perfect (Cameron and van Staveren, 1988). All methods suffer from measurement error. Both systematic and random errors, and the scope of error, differ between the various methods and between various populations; for example between lean and obese people, and between different age groups. Sources of error include under-reporting of food intake, incorrectly estimated portion sizes, and missing or inaccurate nutrient data in food composition tables. For all methods it is important that the measurement error or variability of the method is not too large relative to the actual variability in intake between individuals.

The consumption of specific food groups, for example snacks, is often assessed to evaluate intake with regard to a healthy food pattern. This chapter presents a brief overview of problems with respect to eating behaviour in children and the measurement of food intake.

Eating behaviour in children

An important factor influencing the general health and well-being of an individual is their pattern of food consumption. Unhealthy meal patterns have been implicated in obesity, cholesterol lipoprotein levels, glucose metabolism, plasma hormones, caloric density to energy intake, and nutrient utilization. For example, individuals who consume two or fewer meals daily have been reported to be significantly less healthy and to weigh more than those consuming five or more meals daily.

Methods of dietary assessment

Dietary assessment methods can be divided into those that assess current diet (consisting of records and 24-hour recalls), and those that assess habitual diet (diet histories and food frequency questionnaires). The energy intake data derived from these methods, combined with analytical data from food composition tables or chemical analysis, provide individual nutrient intake. In addition, a number of biological indicators of dietary exposure have been developed, for example, protein in urine, and fatty acids in fat tissue (Kok and van't Veer, 1991; Willett, 1998).

The mode of the report and the characteristics of the respondent, such as their age and culture, also determine the quality of the data collected by these methods (Carbone, Campbell and Hones-Morreale, 2002; Wilson and Lewis, 2004). Modes of self-reporting include face-to-face interviews, telephone interviews, food diaries and records administered by computer or by tape. Not every mode is suitable for all studies. The best mode of self-reporting depends on the research question and on the study population. For instance, if only a limited number of respondents in a population are literate, a diary is not a good choice. Similarly, in remote areas, face-to-face methods are cheaper and more practical. The use of computerized interviews might also lead to less socially desirable answers and result in better estimates of energy intake.

Selecting a method to measure food intake should be based on the type of information that is required, whether it be information required about an individual or group intake, food or food groups, all nutrients or only specific ones (Beaton, 1994). For all methods, there are four types of error: random or systematic within-person error, and random or systematic between-person error. Random within-person error occurs, for example, when the method does not account for day-to-day variation of an individual when determining habitual consumption. It also occurs when replicate measurements cancel out random within-person error. Systematic within-person error may be caused when a person under- or overestimates their food intake; for example, if an important food is not included in a questionnaire. Repeated measurements do not decrease this type of error, which is distributed randomly among individuals. As an overestimation by some individuals is counterbalanced by underestimation by others, the estimated mean intake is consequently not biased. However, this type of error affects precision and widens the distribution artificially. Increasing the number of subjects or replicate measurements may improve precision, but not the validity of estimates for the percentage of undernourished subjects. Systematic between-person error is caused by systematic within-person error that is not randomly distributed among individuals; for example, socially desirable answers provided by groups of people. As a consequence, the mean intake is not estimated correctly, nor is the percentage of undernourished persons.

Assessment of energy intake

There is considerable variation in energy intake from day to day (Willet, 1998). Therefore, one single recall or record does not represent a person's habitual energy intake. The number of days required to assess individual energy intake accurately depends on the within-person variability of intake, derived from information over at least two days. The simple formula of Beaton *et al.* (1979) can be used to calculate the required number of days from within-person variation. This formula is $n = (Z*CVw/D_0)^2$ where n is the number of days required, Z is the normal deviate for the percentage of time the measured value should be within a specified limit, CVw is the within-person coefficient of variation and D_0 is the specified limit. For example, if the CVw is 33 per cent, $n = (1.96*33\%/20\%)^2 = 10$ days. Thus, the number of days necessary to estimate a person's energy intake within 20 per cent will be 10 days. However, if individuals need only to be classified according to their intake, fewer days would be sufficient. For example, when monitoring individuals who lose body weight, assessing changes in energy intake is more relevant than determining absolute intakes.

Under- and over-reporting

To assess the validity of a method it is important to know whether there is a linear or a non-linear relationship between true and reported consumption; that is whether there is differential or non-differential misclassification. If under-reporting is linear to the level of intake, serious bias in estimates of health risks can occur, but it will still be possible to rank individuals according to their energy intake or to assess changes in intake. On the other hand, if under-reporting is non-linear, it will not be possible to rank properly. In general, self-reports are valid means of identifying associations between intake and disease or health. However, these methods cannot determine the actual level of consumption, which makes it difficult to set sensible limits for acceptable intakes or to determine whether intakes meet recommended daily allowances (Beaton, 1994).

Isotope and biochemical markers

It is difficult to determine whether self-reports underestimate or overestimate actual intake, because gold standards against which assessment techniques can be validated are lacking. Energy requirements assessed by the doubly labelled water method (Schoeller, Bandini and Dietz, 1990) are considered the gold standard to assess energy intake. However, the use of the doubly labelled water methodology depends on the premise of energy balance; that is, energy intake equals energy expenditure when subjects are in energy balance (Johnson, Driscoll and Goran, 1996). In addition, because this method requires the costly oxygen-18 isotope and isotope ratio mass spectrometry, its use is limited in large-scale epidemiological studies. Accordingly, the doubly labelled water methodology is primarily employed in validation studies performed in only a small number of subjects.

Predictive equations for basal metabolic rate (based on sex, age, weight or height, or on all these factors) can be used to identify persons whose self-reported energy intakes fall below some physiologically plausible cut-off. This method is easy and inexpensive, but predictive equations may leave out some population subgroups, include activity-related energy expenditure, and identify only extremes of reporting error (Korner *et al.*, 2002).

As a consequence, often only so-called convergent validity can be determined by comparing one method with another. There are three sources of error when comparing results of dietary assessments with biochemical reference standards: (1) the difference between the dietary assessment and the true intake; (2) the effects of digestion, absorption, uptake, utilization, metabolism, excretion and homeo-static mechanisms, all of which impact on the relationship between the amount ingested and the biochemical measurement; and (3) the error associated with the biochemical assay itself (Nelson, 1997). Therefore, a high correlation between two methods does not necessarily mean that a method is valid, since errors of methods are often related; for example, when they both suffer from under-reporting (Willet, 1998).

Underestimation of energy intake

Underestimation of energy intake is more common than overestimation. Schoeller *et al.* (1990) suggested that the reason for under-reporting is that people report their intakes closer to perceived norms than to actual intakes. The results of a large number of validation studies indicate that this occurs between individuals and populations. The average for under-reporting is about 20 per cent (Black *et al.*, 1993); however differences of only 10 per cent by three-day records have been reported in 269 young, lean and motivated subjects (De Vries *et al.*, 1994). As the extent of under-reporting is not necessarily the same for all subjects, it is not a valid option to correct estimated energy consumption by applying a specific factor.

In particular, this under-reporting of energy intake may vary by participants' characteristics. Gender, age and weight status are all predictors of under-reporting. For example, females, older and overweight people are associated with under-reporting energy intake. Other traits that can influence the accuracy of reporting include income, education, social desirability, body image, history of dieting or restrained eating, and depression (Korner *et al.*, 2002).

Obese people tend to report their energy intake more towards that of lean people. In a study of obese subjects by Goris, Westerterp-Platenga and Westerterp (2000), both undereating (a change in body mass over the recording period) and selective under-reporting of food intakes accounted for 37 per cent of under-reporting. Heitmann and Lissner (1995) also found that obese men and women selectively under-report their intakes of fatty foods and foods rich in carbohydrate. The degree of obesity is proportional to the degree of underestimation of energy intake. In addition, individual differences tend to increase as absolute energy values increase, which confirms that subjects who eat more tend to have greater day-to-day variation in food and energy intake (Hise *et al.*, 2002). Such reporting errors consequently confound the ability of researchers to determine habitual energy intakes in overweight and obese individuals.

Underestimation of energy intake may be due to under-reporting or undereating. Undereating could be tracked by measuring body weights during the period of reporting food intake.

Some foods and nutrients are more under-reported than others (Goris and Westerterp, 2000; Heitmann, Lissner and Osler, 2000), but studies are not consistent in the types foods and nutrients that are selectively underestimated. Some studies report underestimation of fat intake, others of carbohydrates, alcohol or specific foods such as snacks. It is also suggested that healthy foods, such as vegetables and fruit, are often overestimated.

When self-reports are repeated in the same subjects, underestimation increases (Goris, Meijer and Westerterp, 2001). This might be a problem, for example when changes in intake are monitored. However, it has also been shown that results improve when subjects are confronted with their own results of underestimation or when they are told that their intake is checked by another method.

In some cultures under-reporting is more prevalent than in others. This could be due to differences in food patterns between populations. It is assumed that regular patterns are easier to recall than patterns with a large variability. Also, social acceptability could play a role. Reporting could be more reliable in populations where unhealthy food habits are more accepted. In the Seneca study, for example, a better relative validity of reporting of alcohol intake was found for the southern European centres than for the northern (van Staveren, Burema and Livingstone, 1996).

Underestimation of portion sizes may be a reason for underestimation of energy intake (Young and Nestle, 1995). Underestimation may be very large, and occurs in all populations. However, portion sizes are also often overestimated. In addition, systematic bias in reporting portion sizes is mentioned; that is small portions are overestimated and large portions are underestimated. Estimations of portion sizes may be improved by the use of food models, weighing of portions, or training in estimating portions.

Measurement in children

There is a growing emphasis by clinicians and researchers on the lifestyle behaviours of children because of the relationship between these behaviours and adulthood diseases such obesity, cardiovascular disease and osteoporosis (Wilson and Lewis, 2004). Any method that requires young children to report their own intake is vulnerable to error because cognitive aspects influence the accuracy of dietary reporting. Compared with adults, children have limited cognitive ability to record or remember their diets, especially in the case of a long interval between consumption and measurement. Children also have difficulty remembering quantities and have less knowledge of food and how the foods are prepared. In addition, they change their food patterns more rapidly (Baranowski and Dome, 1994; Wilson and Lewis, 2004).

Many studies have used one or both parents as a proxy for reporting their children's food intake, or a combined child and parent reporting protocol, especially for children under 10 years of age (Weber *et al.*, 2004). Reports by parents are not always reliable as they are not able to report a child's out-of-home eating (Livingstone and Robson, 2000). In addition, as increasingly often both parents work out of home, it will be more difficult to achieve accurate parental reports of children's eating. Another limitation of parents' reporting is the over-reporting of food intakes and under-reporting of weight of the children, which may occur intentionally to portray their child as eating well and being healthy (Ponza *et al.*, 2004). However, studies which compared parent's reports of their young children's intakes with estimates of energy expenditure determined by the doubly labelled water method showed good agreement (Hill and Davies, 2001).

It is thought that estimation of portion sizes is beyond the intellectual capacity of children. Although training may improve estimations, it has been shown that 35–50 per cent of the children's estimates did not correspond with parental reports (Livingstone and Robson, 2000). The use of training in portion size estimation associated with direct observation of the intake of children can improve the accuracy of their self-reported recalls (Weber *et al.*, 2004).

Bandini *et al.* (2003) found that errors in reported energy intake increased with age for 25 of the 28 girls studied, suggesting that age influences the accuracy of energy intake measurement in adolescents. In an overview of validation studies in children using energy requirements estimated by the doubly labelled water method, Livingstone and Robson (2000) showed that under-reporting increases with age, that obese children under-report more than their lean counterparts, and that some dietary survey methods applied in specific age groups might deal better with under-reporting than others. Furthermore, studies have shown that food intake assessment methods developed for adults do not necessarily apply in adolescents. For example, a study by Droop *et al.* (1995) compared a food frequency questionnaire developed for adults (Feunekes *et al.*, 1993) to assess the intake of energy, total fat, fatty acids and cholesterol in 15-year-old adolescents, with food intake determined by a diet history. The results suggested that, although the adolescents reported the same food groups as the adults, and could be classified well according to their intake, they provided much higher estimates than the adults.

Although adolescents have a relatively better cognitive ability and more knowledge about food than younger children, other factors influence their self-reports, such as less structured food patterns and out-of-home eating. In addition, the meaning of food to children changes as they get older. Initially food satisfies hunger, but later it becomes more a means of self-expression (Bandini *et al.*, 2003). Snacks, carbonated beverages, coffee and tea make up a substantial portion of children's and adolescents' diets, thereby necessitating separate categories for these specific foods in food frequency questionnaires (Johnson, Wardle and Griffith, 2002; Rockett, Wolf and Colditz, 1995). Also, it has been established that the reproducibility of food frequency questionnaires decreases with large intervals. Turconi *et al.* (2003) obtained good correlation between their measures of self-administered questionnaire with an interval of seven days, whereas Rockett, Wolf and Colditz (1995) demonstrated a poor correlation with a one-year interval, indicating low reproducibility of the instrument in study. The results might be explained by the large variation in eating patterns by this group as a result of social or physiological influences.

Other serious problems such as the widespread preoccupation and low satisfaction with body appearance may lead to an increase in unhealthy and extreme methods for weight loss, false concerns about weight-related issues and an increase in the prevalence of eating disorders (McKnight Investigators, 2003; Neumark-Sztainer, 2003). Adolescents with eating disorders can underestimate or overestimate their food intake, for example in those that suffer from bulimia or anorexia nervosa, respectively.

The ratio of the within-person variance of children is generally larger for older children than for younger children and adults. Therefore, more days are often needed to assess intake of older children. However, for specific populations or specific nutrients, within-person variation could be smaller, and number of reporting days could be reduced. This could decrease the burden considerably for participants and experimenters. Fat intake assessed by three-day and four-day estimated food records was compared in 167 children with cystic fibrosis (De Vries, 2003). The within-person variation in their fat intake was 25 per cent, which is less than that of children reported by Willet (1998). Only 0.5 per cent of the children had deviations of more than 20 per cent in fat intake between estimates by three- and four-day records.

In choosing an appropriate method for children, practical aspects might also play a role. An easy method to apply in young children is a 24-hour recall by telephone. This method was administered in 60 children aged five and six years (De Vries, 2003), and interviews took on average 10 minutes. Eighty per cent of the parents were satisfied with this method, and preferred a telephone interview to a personal interview. Energy intake on a group level matched energy requirements.

Improvement of methods

It must be stressed that measurement error of methods could be reduced by practical improvements such as the use of computers. Issues of concern in surveys are incomplete time sampling, poor estimation of portion sizes and recall bias. The use of strictly standardized procedures for sampling, interviewer qualification and training, and quality control is needed to prevent or minimize errors. To assess portion sizes, a picture book or training in estimation of portion sizes is recommended. To improve the validity of food frequency questionnaires and diet records for estimating energy intake, there needs to be an appropriate list of foods that reflects the foods preferred by specific groups, such as children and overweight people, and adequate portion sizes according to the age group. Other questions about the frequency with which respondents prepare the meal themselves or for others in their house, or how often they have a ready-made dinner such as a 'TV dinner', might be useful to evaluate their food pattern.

Conclusions

There are several methods available to assess eating behaviour and food intake in children. The number of days needed for assessment depends upon the method used and the study population involved. Under-reporting is common, especially in the obese. Therefore, it is recommended that other indicators of energy intake be included, such as body weight, height, energy expenditure and physical activity. For children, the method chosen should be adapted to age and food patterns. For adolescents, it is very important that any discrepancies between their perceived and real body image are taken into account.

Future directions for energy intake measures should include larger sample sizes, more diverse populations, additional biomarkers and a wider array of psychosocial measures to elucidate their relationship with under- or over-reporting energy intake.

References

Bandini, L.G., Must, A., Cyr, J., Anderson, S.E., Spadano, J.L. and Dietz W. (2003) 'Longitudinal changes in the accuracy of reported energy intake in girls 10–15 y of age', *American Journal of Clinical Nutrition*, 78: 480–4.

Baranowski, T. and Dome, S.B. (1994) 'A cognitive model of children's reporting of food intake', *American Journal of Clinical Nutrition*, 59(Suppl): S212–17.

Beaton, G.H. (1994) 'Approaches to analyses of dietary data: relationship between planned analyses and choice of methodology', *American Journal of Clinical Nutrition*, 59(Suppl): S253–61.

Beaton, G.H., Milner, J., Corey, P., McGuire, V., Cousins, M., Stewart, E., de Aamos, M., Hewitt, D., Grambsch, P.V., Kassim, N. and Little, J.A. (1979) 'Sources of variance in 24-hour dietary recall data: implications for nutrition study design and interpretation', *American Journal of Clinical Nutrition*, 32: 2546–9.

Black, A.E., Prentice, A.M., Goldberg, G.R., Jebb, S.A., Bingham, S.A., Livingstone, M.B.E. and Coward, W.A. (1993) 'Measurements of total energy expenditure provide insights into the validity of dietary measurements of energy intake', *Journal of the American Dietetic Association*, 93: 572–9.

Cameron, M.E. and van Staveren, W.A. (1998) *Manual on Methodology for Food Consumption Studies*, Oxford: Oxford University Press.

Carbone, E.T., Campbell, M.K. and Hones-Morreale, L. (2002) 'Use of cognitive interview techniques in the development of nutrition surveys and interactive nutrition messages for low-income population', *Journal of the American Dietetic Association*, 102: 690–6.

De Vries, J.H.M. (2003) 'How to measure energy intake in children and adults', in G. Medeiros-Neto, A. Halpern, C. Bouchard (eds) *Progress in Obesity Research*, London: John Libbey, pp. 108–22.

De Vries, J.H., Zock, P.L., Mensink, R.P. and Katan, M.B. (1994) 'Underestimation of energy intake by 3-d records compared with energy intake to maintain body eight in 269 non-obese adults', *American Journal of Clinical Nutrition*, 60: 855–60.

Droop, A., Feunekes, G.I.J., Ham, E., Osendarp, S., Burema, J. and van Staveren, W.A. (1995) 'Vetinneming van adolescenten. Validering van een voedselfrequentievragenlijst die de inneming van vet, vetzuren en cholesterol meet' (in Dutch), *Tijdschr Soc Gezondheidz*, 73: 57–63.

Feunekes, G.I.J., van Staveren, W.A., de Vries, J.H.M., Burema, J. and Hautvast, J.G.A.J. (1993) 'Relative and biomarker-based validity of a food frequency questionnaire estimating intake of fats and cholesterol', *American Journal of Clinical Nutrition*, 58: 489–96.

Goris, A.H., Meijer, E.P. and Westerterp, K.R. (2001) 'Repeated measurement of habitual food intake increases under-reporting and induces selective under-reporting', *British Journal of Nutrition*, 85: 629–34.

Goris, A.H.C. and Westerterp, K.R. (2000) 'Improved reporting of habitual food intake after confrontation with earlier results on food reporting', *British Journal of Nutrition*, 83: 363–9.

Goris, A.H.C., Westerterp-Platenga, M.S. and Westerterp, K. (2000) 'Undereating and underrecording of habitual food intake and exercise in obese men: selective underrecording of fat intake', *American Journal of Clinical Nutrition*, 71: 130–4.

Heitmann, B.L. and Lissner, L. (1995) 'Dietary under-reporting by obese individuals – is it specific or non-specific?', *British Medical Journal*, 311: 986–9.

Heitmann, B.L., Lissner, L. and Osler, M. (2000) 'Do we eat less fat, or just report so?', *International Journal of Obesity and Related Metabolic Disorders*, 24: 435–42.

Hill, R.J. and Davies, O.S. (2001) 'The validity of self-reported energy intake as determined using the doubly labelled water technique', *British Journal of Nutrition*, 85: 415–30.

Hise, M.E., Sullivan, D.K., Jacobsen, D.J., Johnson, S.L., and Donnelly, J.E. (2002) 'Validation of energy intake measurements determined form observer-recorded food records and recall methods compared with the doubly labeled water method in overweight and obese individuals', *American Journal of Clinical Nutrition*, 75: 263–7.

Hoek, A.C., Luning, P.A., Stafleu, A. and de Graaf, C. (2004) 'Food-related lifestyle and health attitudes of Dutch vegetarians, non-vegetarians consumers of meat substitutes, and meat consumers', *Appetite*, 42: 265–72.

Johnson, R.K., Driscoll, P. and Goran, M.I. (1996) 'Comparison of multiple-pass 24-hour recall estimates of energy intake with total energy expenditure determined by the doubly labeled water method in young children', *Journal of the American Dietetic Association*, 96: 1140–4.

Johnson, F., Wardle, J. and Griffith, J. (2002) 'The adolescent food habits checklist: reliability and validity of a measure of healthy eating behaviour in adolescents', *European Journal of Clinical Nutrition*, 56: 644–9.

Kok, F.J. and van't Veer, P. (1991) 'Overview of dietary markers of intake', in F.J. Kok, P. van't Veer (ed.) *Biomarkers of Dietary Exposure*, London: Smith-Gordon, pp. 27–36.

Korner, N.K., Patterson, R.E., Neuhouser, M.L., Lampe, J.W., Beresford, S.A. and Prentice, R.L. (2002) 'Participant characteristics associated with errors in self-reported energy intake from the Women's Health Initiative food frequency questionnaire', *American Journal of Clinical Nutrition*, 76: 766–73.

Livingstone, M.B.E. and Robson, P.J. (2000) 'Measurement of dietary intake in children', *Proceedings of the Nutrition Society*, 59: 279–93.

McKnight Investigators (2003) 'Risk factors for the onset of eating disorders in adolescent girls: results of the McKnight longitudinal risk factor study', *American Journal of Psychiatry*, 160: 248–54.

Nelson, M. (1997) 'The validation of dietary assessment', in B.M. Margetts, M. Nelson (eds) *Design Concepts in Nutritional Epidemiology*, 2nd edition, New York: Oxford University Press, pp. 252–4.

Neumark-Sztainer, D. (2003) 'Obesity and eating disorder prevention: an integrated approach?', *Adolescent Medicine*, 14: 159–73.

Nicklas, T.A., Demory-Luce, D., Yang, S.J., Baranowski, T., Zakeri, I. and Berenson, G. (2004) 'Children's food consumption patterns have changed over two decades (1973–1994): the Bogalusa Heart Study', *Journal of the American Dietetic Association*, 104: 1127–40.

Ponza, M., Devaney, B., Ziegler, P., Reidy, K. and Squatrito, C. (2004) 'Nutrient intakes and food choices of infants and toddlers participating in WIC', *Journal of the American Dietetic Association*, 104(Suppl 1): S71–9.

Rockett, H.R.H., Wolf, A.M. and Colditz, G.A. (1995) 'Development and reproducibility of a food frequency questionnaire to assess diets of older children and adolescents', *Journal of the American Dietetic Association*, 95: 336–40.

Schoeller, D.A. (2003) 'How accurate is self-reported dietary energy intake?', *Nutrition Review*, 48: 373–9.

Schoeller, D.A., Bandini, L.G. and Dietz, W.H. (1990) 'Inaccuracies in self-reported intake identified by comparison with the doubly labelled water method', *Canadian Journal of Physiology and Pharmacology*, 68: 941–9.

van Staveren, W.A., Burema, J. and Livingstone, B.E.M. (1996) 'Evaluation of the dietary history method used in the SENECA study', *European Journal of Clinical Nutrition*, 50(Suppl 2): S47–55.

Turconi, G., Celsa, M., Rezzani, C., Biino, G., Sartirana, M.A. and Roggi, C. (2003) 'Reliability of a dietary questionnaire on food habits, eating behaviour and nutritional knowledge of adolescents', *European Journal of Clinical Nutrition*, 57: 753–63.

Weber, J., Lytle, L., Gittelsohn, J., Cunningham-Sabo, L., Heller, K., Anliker, J.A., Stevens, J., Hurley, J. and Ring, K. (2004) 'Validity of self-reported dietary intake at school meals by American Indian children: the Pathways Study', *Journal of the American Dietetic Association*, 104: 746–52.

Willet, W. (1998) *Nutritional Epidemiology*, 2nd edition, New York: Oxford University Press.

Wilson, A.M.R. and Lewis, R.D. (2004) 'Disagreement of energy and macronutrient intakes estimated from a food frequency questionnaire and 3-day diet record in girls 4 to 9 years of age', *Journal of the American Dietetic Association*, 104: 373–8.

Young, L.R. and Nestle, M. (1995) 'Portion sizes in dietary assessment: issues and policy implications', *Nutrition Review*, 53: 149–58.

10 Physical activity behaviour in children and the measurement of physical activity

L.M. Tomson, T.F. Cuddihy, M. Davidson and R.P. Pangrazi

Introduction

Physical activity and children's health

A significant body of research supports the need for activity and health-related fitness in the lives of youth (Rowland, 1990). Given the substantial increase in obesity among children and adolescents (Magarey, Daniels and Boulton, 2001), physical activity has an important role in helping to combat this serious problem. If lifestyle changes are to be made, physical activity for overweight and obese children should be provided in a setting that is enjoyable and capable of engendering a positive experience (Pangrazi, Corbin and Welk, 1996).

Physical activity is generally defined as bodily movement that is produced by the contraction of skeletal muscle and that substantially increases energy expenditure (Bouchard, 1990; US Department of Health and Human Services, 1996). Therefore, physical activity is an all-encompassing term that includes exercise, sports, dance and leisure activities. In contrast, exercise is commonly undertaken with the intention of developing health and/or physical fitness (Corbin, Pangrazi and Frank, 2000). Physical educators have an important role to play in helping young people to enjoy physical activity and appreciate the benefits of regular participation in activity. This should include attempts to maximize physical activity during the school day to counteract long periods of sitting and inactivity. Teachers and other professionals could also encourage students to develop habitual patterns of physical activity out of school hours (Ernst, Pangrazi and Corbin, 1998).

In Australia, the costs of sedentary living amount to nearly $400 million annually (Bauman *et al.*, 2002). Inactivity among children is a major concern given the near doubling in the prevalence of overweight children between 1985 and 1995 and the more than tripling of the prevalence of obesity in the same period of time (Magarey, Daniels and Boulton, 2001).

One of the major concerns regarding childhood obesity and low levels of physical activity is the predisposition to associated health risk factors. The benefits of physical activity in childhood are numerous. Children who are physically active indicate 'healthier' values on measures such as heart disease risk factors (Raitakari *et al.*, 1994; Sallis *et al.*, 1998; Vaccaro and McMahon, 1989; Vandongen *et al.*, 1995), blood pressure (Dwyer and Gibbons, 1994; Vandongen *et al.*, 1995), total body weight (Epstein *et al.*, 1982; Lazarus *et al.*, 2000; National Health and Medical Research Council, 1997; US Department of Health and Human Services, 1996) and lower levels of total blood cholesterol in conjunction with increased levels of high density lipoprotein (Newman, Freedman and Voors, 1986).

Long-term benefits of a physically active childhood may include the increased likelihood of maintaining a physically active lifestyle through adolescence and into adulthood (Raitakari *et al.*, 1994). Unfortunately, the incorporation of an adequate level of physical activity in a child's life is now becoming even more challenging because of technological advances in society that greatly reduce the opportunity and desire for physical activity (Pangrazi, 2001).

How much physical activity is enough?

As many children are less inclined to voluntarily select continuous vigorous physical activity, activity recommendations are generally defined in terms of the volume of activity (Pangrazi, Corbin and Welk, 1996). The recommendation for at least 60 minutes of daily activity for children and youth (ADHA, 2004a,b) is higher than the 30 minutes per day activity recommendation for adults. Generic adult physical activity recommendations are based primarily on the minimal activity energy expenditure necessary to maintain general health and fitness but predominantly to maintain cardiorespiratory or aerobic fitness. However, it is important that children and youth gain experience in all areas of physical activity and for all components of health-related physical fitness, not limited to aerobic or cardiovascular fitness. For further detail regarding physical activity recommendations for children, readers are encouraged to see the National Association for Sport and Physical Education document authored by Corbin and Pangrazi (2004). The following are guidelines for physical activity for children (ADHA, 2004a).

1 Primary school children should accumulate a minimum of 60 minutes and up to several hours of age-appropriate physical activity on all or most days. Children become less active as they mature, so assuring that youngsters receive 60 minutes a day accounts for a likely decrease in activity levels as they age.
2 Each day, children should be involved in 10–15 minutes of moderate to vigorous activity. This activity should alternate with brief periods of rest and recovery. The natural movement pattern of children is an intermittent style of all-out activity that alternates with periods of rest and recovery. Research shows that bouts of intermittent physical activity (alternating periods of vigorous activity and rest) mirror the release of growth hormone (Bailey *et al.*, 1995). Continuous moderate to vigorous physical activity periods lasting more than five minutes without rest or recovery are rare among children prior to age 13. Because typical activities of children involve sporadic bursts of energy, a greater time involvement rather than a greater intensity of continuous

involvement is recommended. Several (three to six or more) activity sessions spaced throughout the day may be necessary to accumulate adequate activity time for primary school children. Some of these periods should be 10–15 minutes or more in length, alternating intermittent activity and rest within this time period.

3 For adolescents, the guidelines are similar (ADHA, 2004a; Sallis and Patrick, 1994: 318). The major difference is that longer sessions of moderate to vigorous activity are recommended. The guidelines state: 'Adolescents should engage in three or more sessions per week of activities that last 20 minutes or more and require moderate to vigorous levels of exertion.' This is a period of rapid growth and there is evidence to show that alternating aerobic activities with strength and flexibility activities allows youngsters to rest between aerobic intervals and, maybe more importantly, optimizes growth (Pangrazi, Corbin and Welk, 1996).

A common activity target for adult physical activity is the accumulation of 10,000 steps per day (Hatano, 1993); however step goals for children have not yet been established but are likely to be higher (Cuddihy and Michaud-Tomson, 2003). Data show that there is no significant change in children's activity levels from grade 1 to grade 7, but overweight/obese children have a lower step count (recorded by pedometers) than children of normal weight (Tudor-Locke *et al.*, 2004). Given the worldwide obesity epidemic it may be reasonable to set minimum physical activity standards (step counts) linked to the health-related criterion of 'avoidance of overweight/obesity' (Cuddihy and Michaud-Tomson, 2002).

The data illustrated in Table 10.1 indicate that the minimum recommended number of steps/day for girls and boys is 12,000 and 15,000 respectively. In terms of time, the step counts translate to about 120 minutes of daily activity for girls and 150 minutes for boys.

Another way to consider the question 'how much physical activity is enough?' (or how many steps are sufficient?) is to use a 'healthy steps range'. For example, if we use the range from the 20th to the 80th percentile of step data collected on Australian primary school children (Cuddihy and Michaud-Tomson, 2004), this implies that males should be in the range of 11,000–17,000 steps per day and females should be in the range of 9,000–14,100 steps per day. The difference between boys and girls in recommended steps reminds us that weight status has determinants other than physical activity, such as genetics and energy intake (amount and quality).

Children's physical activity levels in Australia

Primary school

A recent Australian study using pedometers to directly measure physical activity in primary school children (Cuddihy and Michaud-Tomson, 2001) suggested that about 61 per cent of Australian boys and 23 per cent of Australian girls are

Table 10.1 Steps/day for youth, stratified by weight status (including mean ± SD)

Age	Normal weight child steps/day (± SD)	Overweight/obese child steps/day (± SD)
Girls		
6	13,246 (3,122)	10,388 (3,016)
7	13,421 (3,843)	11,530 (2,317)
8	12,210 (2,357)	10,795 (2,993)
9	13,445 (2,869)	11,136 (3,491)
10	12,290 (3,105)	11,217 (2,678)
11	13,625 (2,899)	10,539 (3,140)
12	13,405 (2,104)	10,612 (2,117)
Boys		
6	17,548 (1,580)	12,886 (2,610)
7	16,878 (2,469)	13,796 (3,731)
8	16,939 (2,138)	14,290 (3,067)
9	16,520 (3,184)	14,172 (4,067)
10	15,118 (4,203)	12,552 (3,318)
11	16,707 (4,179)	13,296 (2,807)
12	17,074 (2,904)	12,342 (3,440)

achieving the recommended amount of daily physical activity for children (Pan-grazi, Corbin and Welk, 1996). The mean daily step count for boys ($n = 304$) was 14,415 and for girls ($n = 303$) was 11,805 (Vincent *et al.*, 2003). This amounts to about 144 minutes of daily activity for boys and 118 minutes for girls (Cuddihy, van der Bruggen and Pangrazi, 2003).

Results of the assessment of physical activity using pedometers (number of steps per day) with 758 boys and 774 girls in four Queensland schools showed no decline in physical activity levels between grades 1 and 7; in fact a trend of rising levels is noticeable. Males take significantly more steps per day than females at all grade levels. At the 20th percentile, the median steps per day for girls are 9,000 and for boys 11,000. At the 80th percentile, median steps per day for girls are 14,000 and for boys are 17,000.

In another study of 112 grade 5 and 6 children from four Melbourne state primary schools, activity was quantified via accelerometers. The mean time spent in moderate physical activity was 118 minutes per day (which equates to approximately 11,800 steps), and moderate to vigorous activity averaged 16 minutes per day (or about 2000 steps) (Salmon, Telford and Crawford, 2002).

Secondary school

In a study of boys ($n = 297$) in grades 8, 9 and 10, pedometer measures for at least five days over a 10-day period of collection showed that mean daily steps were highly variable and ranged from a minimum daily mean of 5,471 to a maximum of 30,800 steps. The overall mean was 15,500 ± 4,750. There was a significant decline in physical activity from grade 8 to grade 10 (Cuddihy and Michaud-Tomson, 2004). By grade 10, the average movement time was 145 minutes (≈14,500 steps). Of note is that scores for students in the 'most active' group did not decline. In contrast, students in the 'least active' group declined to the extent that their physical activity levels averaged 100 minutes per day less than the 'most active' group (see Figure 10.1). In research on female adolescents, two cohorts were followed for four years, one being a group of grade 8 students and the other a group of grade 10s. The study began with 80 of each grade and finished three years later with 63 remaining in grade 10 and 47 in grade 12. Self-reports showed a significant decline from the 8/9/10 grades to the 11/12 grades in participation in moderate and vigorous physical activity, flexibility and strength activities (Cuddihy *et al.*, 1998).

Physical activity and girls

Commonly, girls' participation in all forms of physical activity, including sport, rapidly declines during their early high school years (Dyer, 1986) with approximately 50 per cent dropping out between the ages of 10 and 14 (Veri and Sahner, 1995). In Australia, 65 per cent of boys as compared with 57 per cent of girls are involved in school-organized sport, club-organized sport or physical activities (ABS, 1998). There was a consistent trend for greater participation in males than females in all age groups, but the difference was marked in the 12–14 and 15–19 year age groups, in which males were 11.2 and 11.3 percentage points higher than females, respectively.

Boys may have an impact on girls' participation in activities at school. Girls do not like to draw attention to themselves and often withdraw from physical education classes and activities that involve participation near or with boys (Australian Sports Commission, 1991). Many girls prefer activities that allow them to work together to improve or to work as a team to accomplish goals (Jaffee and Manzer,

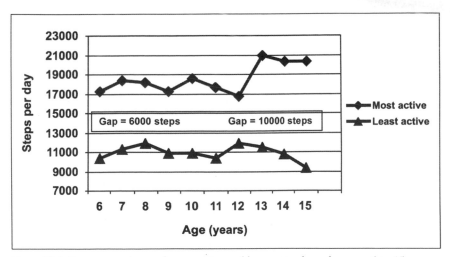

Figure 10.1 Step comparisons of most active and least active boys from age 6 to 15 years.

1992), as opposed to participation in individual competitive activities such as fitness testing (Wiese-Bjornstal, 1997).

Schools as settings for promotion of physical activity

Children spend six hours a day for nearly 40 weeks of the year at school. Thus, it seems logical to utilize this setting for the promotion of physical activity as schools provide both an infrastructure and a context for such programmes (Bauman *et al.*, 2002). Despite the acknowledgment that schools are worthy settings for activity interventions (Australian Health Promoting Schools Association, 1997a,b; National Health and Medical Research Council, 1996; US Department of Health and Human Services, 2000), most interventions to date have been limited to the secondary school setting.

The Child and Adolescent Trial for Cardiovascular Health was an intervention involving US third-graders to reduce or prevent the development of risk factors for cardiovascular disease. A four-part programme was used consisting of health education curricula, a physical education programme, school food service intervention, and a school-wide non-smoking policy. The findings of this study indicated significant improvements in psycho-social determinants such as dietary knowledge, intentions, self-efficacy, usual behaviour, perceived social reinforcement for healthy food choices, and perceived reinforcement and self-efficacy for physical activity (Edmundson *et al.*, 1996). In addition, the intervention was able to achieve a significantly greater volume of moderate to vigorous physical activity in physical education lessons (McKenzie *et al.*, 1996).

In Australia, a physical activity and nutrition intervention for 10- to 12-year-olds was able to change knowledge, fat intake and physical fitness (Vandongen *et al.*, 1995). Recognizing the unique opportunity provided by schools for physical activity promotion, the Australian Federal Government, through the Australian Sports Commission, sought to address declining activity levels by way of an initiative called 'Active Australia'. 'Active Australia' was designed to stimulate and motivate the Australian community to become more involved in a variety of physical activity opportunities in the home, workplace and wider community involving government and non-government agencies at the national, state and local level (Australian Sports Commission, 1997). A core component of the framework was an 'Active Australia Schools Network' with the school environment/ethos, curriculum and community links used to encourage children to develop a physically active lifestyle.

Physical activity out of school hours

Approximately 60 per cent of Australian 5- to 14-year-olds participate in organized sport or physical activity (Australian Bureau of Statistics, 1997). Boys' preferred sports were soccer (20 per cent), swimming (13 per cent), Australian rules football (13 per cent), cricket (10 per cent) and athletics (4 per cent). In contrast, girls' preferred sports included netball (18 per cent), swimming (16 per cent), tennis

(8 per cent), basketball (6 per cent) and athletics (4 per cent). According to parents, 32 per cent of five-year-olds, 69 per cent of 11-year-olds and 58 per cent of 14-year-olds participate in organized sport (Australian Bureau of Statistics, 2000). Despite these levels of participation, Booth *et al.* (1997) contend that fewer than 40 per cent of children surveyed in New South Wales had mastered fundamental movement skills such as running, catching, kicking, striking and throwing. In addition, the after-school period (approximately 3.30–6.30 p.m.) is dominated by sedentary pursuits such as watching television or using the computer/internet.

A study of girls (*n* = 267) in three Queensland primary schools (Davidson, Michaud-Tomson and Cuddihy, 2003) identified sport and bike riding as the most common physical activities. Over 75 per cent of the respondents reported participating in a wide variety of 'other' physical activity (not including sport, swimming or bike riding) outside school time over the four days of data collection, such as dance, karate, horse riding, walking and running.

Active transport to and from school

A major physical activity opportunity for many children is active commuting to and from school, generally walking or cycling. However, a commonly identified barrier to this opportunity to increase physical activity and reduce travel by car is perceived safety (Bauman *et al.*, 2002). Unfortunately, over 60 per cent of children surveyed in Perth (*n* = 2,781) and Melbourne (*n* = 3,198) are driven to school, while 31 per cent and 35 per cent walk in Perth and Melbourne, respectively (Carlin *et al.*, 1997).

Similar patterns of transport to school are evident in North America and Europe. In the USA, transportation surveys show that nearly 50 per cent of 5- to 15-year-olds are driven to school in cars, while about 30 per cent travel by bus and only about 10 per cent walk (US Department of Transportation, Federal Highway Administration, 1997). Sadly, other US research showed that 42 per cent of children being driven to school lived 1 mile (1.6 km) or less from school (McCann and DeLille, 2000). Surveys in Canada present similar results with almost half of the students who completed questionnaires indicating that they travel to school by car (Kowey, 1999). In another study, over 82 per cent of children under 11 years who were within walking distance from their school were transported by car (Go for Green, 1998).

In the United Kingdom car transport to school increased from 16 per cent in 1985/6 to 29 per cent in 1995/7 (Department of the Environment, Transport and the Regions, 1997) with 74 per cent of children travelling less than 1 mile (Osborne and Davis, unpublished). The irony is that, where studies have assessed preference for mode of transport to school, children commonly indicate a preference for walking or cycling (Cleary, 1995).

In Australia, a Perth study revealed that up to 77 per cent of children are driven to school (John, 1999) with a 113 per cent increase in car trips to primary schools in the Perth metropolitan area between 1986 and 1998 (Department for Transport, Western Australian Government, 1999). In Canberra, fewer children (eight to nine years old) were allowed to walk or cycle to school than a generation ago. Younger children were more likely to travel by car and boys were more likely to be allowed to walk or cycle than girls. Schools which had the most walkers or cyclists were located in the middle of a neighbourhood, whereas parents in more affluent areas were more likely to drive children to school (Tranter, 1993). Research refers to a 'car culture' which views modes of travel such as walking and cycling as less attractive than using cars. Beginning at age seven, children are progressively socially conditioned into the car culture (Meaton and Kingham, 1998). Without an established walking and cycling culture in a school, levels of walking and cycling are consistently lower (Wenban-Smith, 1997).

A study of 248 grade 5 children at four schools in Brisbane, Queensland, reinforced that the motor vehicle is the most common form of transport to school (67 per cent) followed by walking (19.8 per cent) and cycling (4.4 per cent). Significantly more girls were driven to school. As in the USA, UK and Canada, a car trip time of five minutes or less was the most common. Ironically, 54 per cent of the parents in the Brisbane survey walked to school when they were children and only 1.6 per cent travelled by car (Ridgewell, 2000).

In work completed by the authors (491 grade 4–7 children), children who walked to school averaged significantly more steps per day than those who travelled by bus or car, and were also more likely to play sport. The impact of walking to school on total steps per day versus all other forms of transport amounted to approximately 3,500 steps, or 30–35 minutes of additional physical activity. This study indicates that walking to school holds real promise as a meaningful way of impacting children's overall physical activity levels.

Monitoring and measuring physical activity levels

Numerous methods have been used to assess physical activity; these vary in usefulness depending on desired precision and accuracy of the technique, the intended use for the data, and those responsible for measurement. A general description of a range of methods follows, including advantages and disadvantages of each method.

Self-report and recall

Self-reports may include diaries completed by the individual, self-administered questionnaires, interviewer questionnaires, and proxy reports completed by parents or teachers. Self-report instruments have the advantages of being cost-effective, user-friendly (Welk and Wood, 2000) and easy to administer with minimal participant burden. Both qualitative and quantitative data can be collected; however, there is a heavy reliance on the accuracy of information provided by the individual.

The self-report technique is more useful in adults (Harro and Riddoch, 2000) with reliability and validity concerns such as subject bias and difficulty for many children in recalling physical activities accurately (Baranowski, 1988; Sallis, 1991;

Sallis *et al.*, 1993; Weston, Petosa and Pate, 1997). A further issue is that both adults and children frequently overestimate their actual activity level. Despite these limitations, Sallis and Saelens (2000) have shown that there are a number of recall instruments that have acceptable reliability and validity when they are used with adolescent and adult populations. Refer to the review of self-report instruments by Matthews (2002) for further detail.

Direct observation

McKenzie (1991) reported that the direct observation technique is highly effective in measuring physical activity levels. An observer logs both the intensity and type of activity performed during short sporadic intervals. Despite being valid and reliable, the approach is labour intensive and time consuming (Kilanowski, Consalvi and Epstein, 1999; Welk and Wood, 2000) even for trained observers. More advanced software programs have helped to enhance data collection, recording and subsequent analysis. A program by Sharpe and Koperwas (2000), marketed as the Behavior Evaluation Strategies and Taxonomies (BEST) system, allows for codes and behaviours to be inserted and defined in a relatively flexible manner.

A number of observation applications are available for use in different settings and with children of different ages. McKenzie (2002) has written a review of nine applications that show acceptable validity and reliability with physical activity codes in these instruments validated against an energy expenditure measure and classified by school and non-school settings. Most of these systems collect data related to frequency, duration, and the amount of time between behaviours (latency).

Two of the more widely used instruments are SOFIT (System for Observing Fitness Instruction Time) and SOPLAY (System for Observing Play and Leisure Activity in Youth) (McKenzie, Sallis and Nadar, 1991; McKenzie *et al.*, 2000). SOFIT measures student physical activity, lesson content and teacher behaviour during physical education classes. Lesson content is categorized as management, fitness, knowledge, skill drills, game play and free play. Despite being useful for the evaluation of the amount of physical activity received in the physical education setting, the instrument does not measure total physical activity while at school.

SOPLAY is designed to examine activity levels of children in different settings. This objective instrument assesses the activity level of groups of people in a designated activity area rather than individuals and is therefore appropriate for use in open environments such as parks, recreational programmes or school playgrounds. SOPLAY uses momentary time sampling, and observation requires mapping the target area to ensure that data is collected from a consistent point.

Systematic observation is an effective technique, but much training and observation time are required. Some would argue that it is only useful in a research context; however, when working with obese youngsters in limited numbers, this approach may be very useful.

Activity monitors

Trost (2001: 32) describes accelerometers as 'second-generation' motion sensors that provide real-time estimates of the frequency, intensity and duration of free-living physical activity. Accelerometers have gained widespread acceptance for the measurement of activity (Freedson and Miller, 2000; Haskell *et al.*, 1993; Melanson and Freedson, 1995; Saris, 1986). There are numerous manufacturers of activity monitors and in uni-axial, bi-axial or tri-axial modes. The integration of time and activity allows a verification of activity level with data stored in the monitor and downloaded to a personal computer for analysis.

An advantage of accelerometers is the inability of participants to tamper with the input; however, a disadvantage is the inability to provide immediate feedback and motivation for the user. Another drawback of the widespread use of activity monitors in the field is their relative expense. The cost of monitors may limit the number of participants who may participate in activity programmes.

Pedometers

Pedometers measure the number of steps a person takes whilst involved in ambulatory activities. Electronic pedometers detect movement through a spring-loaded, counter-balanced mechanism that records vertical acceleration at the hip. Pedometers are more cost-effective than accelerometers or heart rate monitors and are a valid measurement option (Tudor-Locke *et al.*, 2002). Recent advances in technology have significantly improved the accuracy of some pedometers (Bassett *et al.*, 1996; Freedson, 1991; Trost, 2001; Welk and Wood, 2000) and, like accelerometers, the devices are unobtrusive and convenient to use (Gretebeck and Montoye, 1992; Rowlands, Eston and Ingledew, 1997; Sequeira *et al.*, 1995; Welk *et al.*, 2000). Steps recorded by the Yamax Digiwalker pedometers used in a study by Eston, Rowlands and Ingledew (1997) were highly correlated (0.92) with scaled oxygen consumption during treadmill walking/running and unrestricted play activities in 8- to 10-year-old children. Kilanowski, Consalvi and Epstein (1999) also confirmed high validity when working with 12-year-old children and correlations of greater than 0.95 were obtained between electronic pedometer steps per minute and directly observed physical activity.

Validation of the pedometer as a reliable method of collecting data was reported in a comparison of activity levels during recreational activities with classroom activities using a Tritrac accelerometer and direct observation (Children's Activity Rating System, CARS) (Kilanowski, Consalvi and Epstein, 1999). In another study, pedometers were compared with accelerometers, heart rate monitors and oxygen uptake (VO_2) in regulated (walking and jogging) and unregulated activities (hopscotch, throwing, catching and colouring). The pedometer accounted for a greater proportion of the variance in regression analysis than either heart rate or uni-axial accelerometer (Eston, Rowlands and Ingledew, 1998). The pedometer may be best suited to research that identifies physical activity levels in free-living conditions or 'studies in which the goal is to document relative changes in physical activity or to rank order groups of children on physical activity participation' (Trost, 2001).

However, it is important to acknowledge the limitations of pedometers. Pedometers are less accurate when people move slowly (less than 4 km/h) or walk with an uneven gait (Crouter *et al.*, 2003), and they overestimate distance covered at slower speeds and underestimate actual distance at higher speeds (Schneider *et al.*, 2003). Caloric expenditure is also usually overestimated (Crouter *et al.*, 2003). Errors in distance and energy expenditure are not surprising as most pedometers do not account for step length and walking speed differences. A fundamental problem is associated with the ease of registration of counts (steps) associated with extraneous movements that may be unrelated to ambulatory activity. Accumulated duration of physical activity is a relatively accurate pedometer measure because it is not affected by step length or movement speed. This is also an advantage because most activity guidelines are stated in minutes of activity accumulated each day.

Orientation of the pedometer is also an important issue; if not parallel with the vertical plane accuracy is affected. Furthermore, pedometers cannot measure water-based activity, skating, cycling, ice-skating or horse riding. In spite of these limitations, the reasonable cost of pedometers and their potential as a motivational tool for many people, including overweight and obese children, should not be overlooked. Pedometers make it possible to collect data on large numbers of participants because they are relatively inexpensive (Cuddihy, Pangrazi and Michaud-Tomson, 2005).

Heart rate monitors

Heart rate monitors enable the assessment of physical activity levels over extended periods of time with relative ease (Trost, 2001; Welk and Wood, 2000). Heart rate has long been used to monitor the intensity of physical activity over time and store data collected in varying time intervals and later downloaded to a computer. Heart rate monitors can be used in both laboratory and field settings and provide safe training zones for users, including in the context of weight management.

However, physical activity can cause an increase in heart rate without increased energy expenditure (Melanson and Freedson, 1996) and factors such as increased ambient temperature, emotional stress, age and training state all have the potential to impact on heart rate. Heart rate monitors are also unable to distinguish between upper body/static work heart rates compared to lower body aerobic work (Rowlands, Eston and Ingledew, 1997; Saris, 1986), for example weight lifting.

Heart rate monitors primarily respond accurately to aerobic types of activity. Since they focus on the intensity of aerobic activity, they may not be the instrument of choice when working with obese youth. These youngsters may already be opposed to intense activity and perceive it to be quite difficult. In this case, focusing on movement of all types rather than intensity may be more appropriate. In a school setting, some participants do not like to wear the straps around their chest and see them as intrusive or even uncomfortable when worn for a number of hours. Additional considerations for the use of this instrument are the cost, which would be prohibitive for a large number of students, as well as the difficulty in gathering information outside school hours.

References

ABS (Australian Bureau of Statistics) (1997) *Participation in Sport and Physical Activities, Australia, 1995–96,* Canberra: Australian Government Publishing Service.

ABS (Australian Bureau of Statistics) (1998) *Culture and Recreation: Participation in Sport and Physical Activities,* Canberra: Australian Government Publishing Service

ABS (Australian Bureau of Statistics) (2000) *Children's Participation in Cultural and Leisure Activities,* Canberra: Australian Government Publishing Service.

ADHA (Australian Department of Health and Ageing) (2004a) *Australia's Physical Activity Recommendations for 5–12 Year Olds.* Canberra: ADHA.

ADHA (Australian Department of Health and Ageing) (2004b) *Australia's Physical Activity Recommendations for 12–18 Year Olds.* Canberra: ADHA.

Australian Health Promoting Schools Association (1997a) *National Strategy for Health Promoting Schools, 1998–2001,* Sydney: Australian Health Promoting Schools Association.

Australian Health Promoting Schools Association (1997b) *School-based Health Promotion Across Australia. Background Briefing Report no. 1. National Health Promoting Schools Initiative, 1997,* Sydney: Australian Health Promoting Schools Association.

Australian Sports Commission (1991) *Sport for Young Australians: Widening the Gateways to Participation,* Canberra: Australian Sports Commission.

Australian Sports Commission (1997) *Active Australia: A National Participation Framework,* Canberra: Australian Sports Commission.

Bailey, R.C., Olson, J., Pepper, S.L., Porszaz, J., Barstow, T.J. and Cooper, D.M. (1995) 'The level and tempo of children's physical activities: an observational study', *Medicine and Science in Sports and Exercise,* 27: 1033–41.

Baranowski, T. (1988) 'Validity and reliability of self-report measures on physical activity: an information processing perspective', *Research Quarterly for Exercise and Sport,* 59: 314–27.

Bassett, D.R.J., Ainsworth, B.E., Leggett, S.R., Mathien, C.A., Main, J.A., Hunter, D.C. and Duncan, G.E. (1996) 'Accuracy of five electronic pedometers for measuring distance walked', *Medicine and Science in Sports and Exercise,* 28: 1071–7.

Bauman, A., Bellew, B., Vita, P., Brown, W. and Owen, N. (2002) *Getting Australia Active: Towards Better Practice for the Promotion of Physical Activity,* Melbourne: National Public Health Partnership.

Booth, M., Macaskill, P., McLellan, L., Phongsavan, P., Okley, T., Patterson, J. Wright, J., Bauman, A. and Baur, L. (1997) *NSW Schools Fitness and Physical Activity Survey, 1997,* Sydney: NSW Department of Education.

Bouchard, C. (1990) 'Discussion: heredity, fitness and health', in C. Bouchard, R.J. Shephard, T. Stephens, J.R. Sutton, B.D. McPherson (eds) *Exercise, Fitness and Health,* Champaign, IL: Human Kinetics.

Carlin, J.B., Stevenson, M.R., Roberts, I., Bennett, C.M., Gelman, A. and Nolan, T. (1997) 'Walking to school and traffic exposure in Australian children', *Australia New Zealand Journal of Public Health,* 21: 286–92.

Cleary, J. (1995) 'School travel, health and the environment', in M. Gerecke (ed.) *Proceedings of the 8th Velo-City Conference,* Basel: VCC.

Corbin C.B. and Pangrazi, R.P. (2004) *Physical Activity for Children: A Statement of Guidelines for Children Ages 5–12*, Reston, VA: National Association for Sport and Physical Education.

Corbin, C.B., Pangrazi, R.P. and Frank, B.D. (2000) 'Definitions: health, fitness, and physical activity', *Research Digest*, 3(9).

Crouter, S.C., Schneider, P.L., Karabulut, M. and Bassett, D.R., Jr (2003) 'Validity of 10 electronic pedometers for measuring steps, distance, and energy cost', *Medicine and Science in Sports and Exercise*, 35: 1455–60.

Cuddihy, T.F. and Michaud-Tomson, L.M. (2001) 'Children's physical activity level and BMI: effects of age and gender', paper presented at Australasian Society for the Study of Obesity Conference, Gold Coast, Australia.

Cuddihy, T.F. and Michaud-Tomson, L. (2002) 'Children's daily physical activity levels and body composition', paper presented at International Sports Sciences Conference, Hong Kong, China.

Cuddihy, T.F. and Michaud-Tomson, L. (2003) 'The healthy steps per day range for children in Grades 1–7', paper presented at National Physical Activity Conference, Perth, Australia.

Cuddihy, T.F. and Michaud-Tomson, L. (2004) 'The healthy steps range for children aged 6–16', paper presented at Australian Association for Exercise and Sport Science Conference in Brisbane, Australia.

Cuddihy, T., Pangrazi, R.P. and Michaud-Tomson, L. (2005) 'Pedometers: answers to FAQ's from teachers', *Journal of Physical Education, Recreation & Dance*, 76(2): 36–40.

Cuddihy, T. F., Costin, G., Davies, P., Hills, A. and Parker, A. (1998) 'Longitudinal changes in intrinsic motivation and physical activity patterns for adolescent females', paper presented at the Australian Conference of Science and Medicine in Sport, Adelaide, Australia.

Cuddihy, T.F., van der Brugen, C. and Pangrazi, R.P. (2003) 'Accuracy of the Walk-for-Life (LS2505) pedometer at different walking speeds and on different terrain', paper presented at National Physical Activity Conference, Perth, Australia.

Davidson, M.A., Michaud-Tomson, L. and Cuddihy, T.F (2003) 'A comparison of the physical activity levels of girls at state and private primary schools', *ACHPER Healthy Lifestyles Journal*, 50: 7–13.

Department of the Environment, Transport and the Regions (1997) *Transport Statistics Report: National Travel Survey, 1994–1996*, Vancouver, Canada.

Department for Transport, Western Australian Government (1999) *Travelsmart, 2010*, Perth: WA Government.

Dwyer, T. and Gibbons, L.E. (1994) 'The Australian Schools Health and Fitness survey: physical fitness related to blood pressure but not lipoproteins', *Circulation*, 89: 1539–44.

Dyer, K.F. (1986) *Girls' Physical Education and Self-esteem: A Review of Research Resources and Strategies*, Canberra: Commonwealth Schools Commission.

Edmundson, E., Parcell, G.S., Perry, C.L., Feldman, H.A., Smyth, M., Johnson, C.C., Layman, A., Bachman, K., Perkins, T., Smith, K. and Stone, E. (1996) 'The effects of the child and adolescent trial for cardiovascular health intervention on psycho-social determinants of cardiovascular disease risk behavior among third-grade students', *American Journal of Health Promotion*, 10: 217–25.

Epstein, L.H., Wing, R.R., Koeske, R., Ossip, D. and Beck, S. (1982) 'A comparison of lifestyles change and programmed aerobic exercise on weight loss in obese children', *Behaviour Therapy*, 13: 651–65.

Ernst, M.P., Pangrazi, R.P. and Corbin, C.B. (1998) 'Physical education: making a transition toward activity', *Journal of Physical Education, Recreation & Dance*, 69(9): 29–32.

Eston, R.G., Rowlands, A.V. and Ingledew, D.K. (1998) 'Validity of heart rate, pedometry, and accelerometry for predicting the energy cost of children's activities', *Journal of Applied Physiology*, 84: 362–71.

Freedson, P.S. (1991) 'Electronic motion sensors and heart-rate as measures of physical attraction in children', *Journal of School Health*, 6: 215–19.

Freedson, P.O. and Miller, K. (2000) 'Objective monitoring of physical activity using motion sensors and heart rate', *Research Quarterly for Exercise and Sport*, 71: 21–9.

Go for Green (1998) *Go for Green Newsletter*, 2(3). Ontario: Go for Green.

Gretebeck, R.J. and Montoye, H.J. (1992) 'Variability of some objective measures of physical activity', *Medicine and Science in Sports and Exercise*, 24: 1167–72.

Harro, M. and Riddoch, C. (2000) 'Physical activity', in N. Armstrong, W. van Mechelen (eds) *Paediatric Exercise Science and Medicine*, Oxford: Oxford University Press, pp. 77–84.

Haskell, W.L., Yee, M.C., Evans, A. and Irby, P.J. (1993) 'Simultaneous measurement of heart rate and body motion to quantify physical activity', *Medicine and Science in Sports and Exercise*, 25: 109–15.

Hatano, Y. (1993) 'Use of the pedometer for promoting daily walking exercise', *Journal of the International Council for Health, Physical Education and Recreation*, 29: 4–9.

Jaffee, L. and Manzer, R. (1992) 'Girls' perspectives: physical activity and self-esteem', *A Journal for Women's Health Research*, 11: 14–23.

John, G. (1999) 'Travelsmart to school: an innovative approach to influencing travel behaviour', paper presented at WA Division – Institute of Municipal Engineering Conference, Perth, Australia.

Kilanowski, C.A., Consalvi, A. and Epstein, L.H. (1999) 'Validation of an electronic pedometer for measurement of physical activity in children', *Pediatric Exercise Science*, 1: 63–8.

Kowey, B. (1999) 'The journey to school: making it safer by reducing traffic at school sites and increasing pedestrian and driver education opportunities', paper presented at Canadian Multidisciplinary Road Safety Conference XI, Vancouver, Canada.

Lazarus, J., Wake, M., Hesketh, K. and Waters, E. (2000) 'Changes in body mass index in Australian primary school children, 1985–1997', *International Journal of Obesity*, 24: 679–84.

McCann, B. and DeLille, B. (2000) *Mean Streets 2000: Pedestrian Safety, Health and Federal Transportation Spending*, Columbia, SC: Centers for Disease Control and Prevention.

McKenzie, T.L. (1991) 'Observational measures of children's physical activity', *Journal of School Health*, 61: 224–7.

McKenzie, T.L. (2002) 'Use of direct observation to assess physical activity', in G. Welk (ed.) *Physical Activity Assessments for Health-Related Research*, Champaign, IL: Human Kinetics, pp. 179–95.

McKenzie, T.L., Sallis, J.F. and Nadar, P.R. (1991) 'SOFIT: System for Observing Fitness Instruction Time', *Journal of Teaching in Physical Education*, 11: 195–205.

McKenzie, T.L., Nader, P.R., Strikmuller, P.K., Yang, M., Stone, E.J., Perry, C.L., Taylor, W.C., Epping, J.N., Feldman, H.A., Luepker, R.V. and Kelder, S.H. (1996) 'School physical education: effect of the child and adolescent trial for cardiovascular health', *Preventive Medicine*, 25: 423–31.

McKenzie, T.L., Marshall, S.J., Sallis, J.F. and Conway, T.L. (2000) 'Leisure-time physical activity in school environments: an observational study using SOPLAY', *Preventive Medicine*, 30: 70–7.

Magarey, A.M., Daniels, L.A. and Boulton, T.J. (2001) 'Prevalence of overweight and obesity in Australian children and adolescents: reassessment of 1985 and 1995 data against new standard international definitions', *Medical Journal of Australia*, 174: 561–4.

Matthews, C.E. (2002) 'Use of self-report instruments to assess physical activity', in G. Welk (ed.) *Physical Activity Assessments for Health-Related Research*, Champaign, IL: Human Kinetics, pp. 107–23.

Meaton, J. and Kingham, S. (1998) 'Children's perceptions of transport modes: car culture in the classroom?', *World Transport Policy and Practice*, 4: 12–16.

Melanson, E.L., Jr and Freedson, P.S. (1995) 'Validity of the Computer Science and Applications, Inc. (CSA) activity monitor', *Medicine and Science in Sports and Exercise*, 27: 934–40.

Melanson, E.L. and Freedson, P.S. (1996) 'Physical activity assessment: a review of methods', *Critical Reviews in Food Science and Nutrition*, 36: 385–96.

National Health and Medical Research Council (1996) *Effective School Health Promotion: Towards Health Promoting School*, Canberra: AGPS.

National Health and Medical Research Council (1997) *Acting on Australia's Weight: A Strategic Plan for the Prevention of Overweight and Obesity*, Canberra: AGPS.

Newman, W.P., Freedman, D.S., and Voors, A.W. (1986) 'Relation of serum lipoprotein levels and systolic blood pressure to early atherosclerosis. The Bogalusa Heart Study', *New England Journal of Medicine*, 314: 138–44.

Osborne, P. and Davis, A. (unpublished) *Safe routes to school demonstration project*, Bristol: Sustrans.

Pangrazi, R.P. (2001) *Dynamic Physical Education for Elementary School Children*, 13th edition, Sydney: Allyn and Bacon.

Pangrazi, R.P., Corbin, C.B. and Welk, G.J. (1996) 'Physical activity for children and youth', *Journal of Physical Education, Recreation and Dance*, 67: 38–43.

Raitakari, O.T., Porkka, K.V.K., Taimela, S., Telama, R., Tasanen, L. and Viikari, J.S.A. (1994) 'Effects of persistent physical activity and inactivity on coronary risk factors in children and young adults', *American Journal of Epidemiology*, 140: 195–205.

Ridgewell, C. (2000) 'Modal choices for school travel in Brisbane', unpublished thesis, Griffith University.

Rowland, T.W. (1990) *Exercise and Children's Health*, Champaign, IL: Human Kinetics.

Rowlands, A.V., Eston, R.G. and Ingledew, D.K. (1997) 'Measurement of physical activity in children with particular reference to the use of heart rate and pedometry', *Sports Medicine*, 24: 258–72.

Sallis, J.F. (1991) 'Self-report measures of children's physical activity', *Journal of School Health*, 61: 215–19.

Sallis, J. F. and Patrick, K. (1994) 'Physical activity guidelines for adolescents: consensus statement', *Pediatric Exercise Science*, 6: 302–14.

Sallis, J.F. and Saelens, B.E. (2000) 'Assessment of physical activity by self-report: status, limitations, and future directions', *Research Quarterly for Exercise and Sport*, 71: 1–14.

Sallis, J.F., Buono, M.J., Roby, J.J., Micale, F.G. and Nelson, J.A. (1993) 'Seven day recall and other physical activity self-reports in children and adolescents', *Medicine and Science in Sports and Exercise*, 25: 99–108.

Sallis, J.F., Patterson, T.L., Buono, M.J. and Nader, P.R. (1998) 'Relation of cardiovascular fitness and physical activity to cardiovascular disease risk factors in children and adults', *American Journal of Epidemiology*, 127: 933–41.

Salmon, J., Telford, A. and Crawford, D. (2002) 'Assessment of physical activity among primary school aged children: the Children's Leisure Activities Study (CLASS)', *Australasian Epidemiologist*, 9: 10–14.

Saris, W.H.M. (1986) 'Habitual physical activity in children: methodology and findings in health and disease', *Medicine and Science in Sports and Exercise*, 18: 253–63.

Schneider, P.L., Crouter, S.E., Lukajic, O. and Bassett, D.R., Jr (2003) 'Accuracy and reliability of 10 pedometers for measuring steps over at 400-m walk', *Medicine and Science in Sports and Exercise*, 35: 1779–84.

Sequeira, M.M., Rickenbach, M., Wietlisbach, V., Tullen, B. and Schutz, Y. (1995) 'Physical activity assessment using a pedometer and its comparison with a questionnaire in a large population survey', *American Journal of Epidemiology*, 142: 989–99.

Sharpe, T.L. and Koperwas, J. (2000) *Software Assist for Education and Social Science Settings: Behavior Evaluation Strategies and Taxonomies (BEST) and Accompanying Qualitative Applications*, 2nd edition, Thousand Oaks, CA: Sage-Scolari.

Tranter, R. (1993) *Children's Mobility in Canberra: Confinement or Independence?*, Monograph Series No. 7, Canberra: Department of Geography and Oceanography, University College, Australian Defence Force Academy, University of New South Wales.

Trost, S.T. (2001) 'Objective measurement of physical activity in youth: current issues, future directions', *Exercise in Sport Science Reviews*, 29: 32–6.

Tudor-Locke, C., Williams, J.E., Reis, J.P. and Pluto, D. (2002) 'Utility of pedometers for assessing physical activity: convergent validity', *Sports Medicine*, 32: 795–808.

Tudor-Locke, C., Pangrazi, R.P., Corbin, C.B., Rutherford, W.J., Vincent, S.D., Raustorp, A., Michaud-Tomson, L. and Cuddihy, T.F. (2004) 'BMI-referenced standards for recommended pedometer-determined steps/day in children', *Preventive Medicine*, 38: 857–64.

US Department of Health and Human Services (1996) *Physical Activity and Health: A Report of the Surgeon General*, Atlanta, GA: US Department of Health and Human Services, Centers for Disease Control and Prevention, National Center for Chronic Disease Prevention and Health Promotion.

US Department of Health and Human Services (2000) *Healthy People 2010*, 2nd edition, Washington, DC: US Department of Health and Human Services.

US Department of Transportation, Federal Highway Administration (1997) *Our Nation's Travel: 1995 NPTS Early Result Report*, Washington, DC: US Government Printing Office.

Vaccaro, P. and McMahon, A.D. (1989) 'The effects of exercise on coronary heart disease risk factors in children', *Sports Medicine*, 8: 139–53.

Vandongen, R., Jenner, D., Thompson, C., Taggart, A., Spickett, E., Burke, V., Beilin, L., Milligan, R. and Dunbar, D. (1995) 'A controlled evaluation of a fitness and nutrition intervention program on cardiovascular health in 10–12 year old children', *Preventive Medicine*, 24: 9–22.

Veri, M.J. and Sahner, K.P. (1995) *Girls and Women in Sport to be Honored on Thursday*, [online] available from <http://dailybeacon.edu/issues/v68/n14/women.14v.html>.

Vincent, S.D, Pangrazi, R.P., Raustorp, A., Michaud-Tomson, L. and Cuddihy, T.F. (2003) 'Activity levels and body mass index of children in the United States, Sweden and Australia', *Medicine and Science in Sports and Exercise*, 35: 1367–73.

Welk, G.J. and Wood, K. (2000) 'Physical activity assessment in physical education – a practical review of instruments and their use in the curriculum', *Journal of Physical Education, Recreation and Dance*, 71: 44–9.

Welk, G.J., Differding, J.A., Thompson, R., Blair, S.N., Dziura, J, and Hart, P. (2000) 'The utility of the digi-walker step counter to assess daily physical activity patterns', *Medicine and Science in Sports and Exercise*, 32: S481–8.

Wenban-Smith, J. (1997) 'Safe routes to schools', *Transport Report*, 20: 12–13.

Weston, A.T., Petosa, R. and Pate, R.R. (1997) 'Validation of an instrument for measurement of physical activity in youth', *Medicine and Science in Sports and Exercise*, 29: 138–43.

Wiese-Bjornstal, D. (1997) 'Section II: psychological dimensions', in L.K. Bunker (ed.) *The President's Council on Physical Fitness and Sport Report: Physical Activity and Sport in the Lives of Girls*, Washington, DC: President's Council.

11 Environmental factors and physical activity in children

Implications for active transport programmes

J. Yeung, S.C. Wearing and A.P. Hills

Introduction

Childhood obesity represents a serious national and international health problem, with one in four Australian children now classified as overweight or obese. Whereas physical activity has been recognised as an important element in combating childhood obesity, factors governing activity levels in children are poorly understood. Environmental factors, however, appear to play a key role in governing activity levels in communities and, as such, represent an important consideration for interventions designed to increase physical activity in children. Ideally, programmes targeting childhood obesity should encourage all children to be physically active and to provide them with an environment that is conducive to regular physical activity. The development and successful execution of such programmes is predicated on the identification of potential environmental barriers that prevent a physically active lifestyle and promote weight gain.

Although poorly understood, the aetiology of obesity has been considered from a range of perspectives, including genetic, environmental and behavioural factors and their interaction (Crawford and Ball, 2002; Loke, 2002; Maddock, 2004; McGuire *et al.*, 1999; Marti *et al.*, 2004; Ochoa *et al.*, 2004). Although genetic factors have received considerable attention within the literature, they are unlikely to account for the sudden increase in obesity noted worldwide given the relative stability of the gene pool (Jequier, 2002). Therefore, recent research has focused on the role of environmental and behavioural factors in the development of obesity. Whereas most researchers agree that energy balance and hence body weight are regulated phenomena (Jequier and Tappy, 1999), Egger and Swinburn (1997) contend that body fat levels represent a 'settling' rather than 'set' point, and are dependent on biological, behavioural and environmental influences which impact upon adiposity by acting through the mediators of energy intake and energy expenditure. In particular, Swinburn, Egger and Raza (1999) contend that modern individuals struggle against environments that increasingly promote high energy intake and sedentary behaviours. In support of this concept, the built environment has been shown to influence both obesity and physical activity levels at the population level (Burdette and Whitaker, 2004; Frank, Andresen and Schmid,

2004; Maddock, 2004). Thus, one might contend that the major challenge for society, with respect to obesity prevention in children, is to create supportive environments that facilitate opportunities to be physically active which in turn are conducive to the maintenance of a healthy body composition. The aim of this chapter is to present the major environmental issues and challenges associated with promotion of physical activity in children and to provide a specific example of how barriers identified by the ANGELO framework can be modified in the development of a 'Walk-to-School' programme.

Modifications to the environment necessary to afford a shift in activity levels

In reviewing interventions for preventing childhood obesity, Campbell *et al.* (2002) proposed that preventive strategies should encourage both a reduction in sedentary behaviours and a concomitant increase in physical activity. An important challenge is to encourage all children to be physically active and to provide them with an environment that is conducive to regular physical activity (Hills and Cambourne, 2002). Given the diversity of urban and rural settings and the mix of socioeconomic determinants representative of contemporary society, the task may be difficult, but not impossible (Garcia *et al.*, 1995). Ball and Crawford (2003) maintain that it is only by gaining an understanding of these contextual influences that insight necessary to effectively respond to the epidemic of obesity will be developed. The ANGELO framework, first outlined by Swinburn, Egger and Raza (1999), offers a concrete opportunity to assist in the achievement of such an understanding by providing an analysis grid for environments linked to obesity. It is under the auspices of the ANGELO framework that this chapter will highlight the main obesogenic elements within the environment that impact upon intervention strategies designed to promote physical activity in children.

The ANGELO framework – a means of understanding the obesogenic environment

Swinburn, Egger and Raza (1999) propose that the main barriers to the successful development and execution of environmental interventions include the lack of suitable paradigms and tools for understanding and measuring the environment. To assist in the identification of obesogenic factors in the environment they developed the ANGELO framework. As demonstrated in Table 11.1, the framework categorises elements of the environment on the basis of size and type. Individuals interact with multiple settings or 'microenvironments', including homes, schools, workplaces and neighbourhoods and these, in turn, are influenced by broader 'macroenvironments'. Macroenvironmental sectors provide for less control by individuals and include all levels of government, education, health and the food industry. Both micro- and macroenvironments may be further subdivided into physical, economic, political and sociocultural elements.

Table 11.1 Environmental considerations in promoting physical activity as a method to prevent childhood obesity

Size	Environment			
	Physical	Economic	Political	Sociocultural
Micro				
School	Adequate indoor and outdoor spaces and infrastructure Availability of sports equipment and activity-promoting toys Physical activity programmes Adequate teacher training	Costs associated with equipment and infrastructure	School policies on health and physical education programmes Policies regarding traffic congestion and transport Policies regarding recess	School ethos regarding physical activity Teacher attitudes towards physical activity
Home	Sports equipment Sufficient yard space	Parental time Sports equipment costs Membership and game fees	Parental restrictions on activity	Parental attitudes and beliefs towards physical activity Affinity for motorised transport Parent engagement as role models
Neighbourhood	Off-street recreation and sports facilities Safe walking and cycling paths Educational interventions	Funding support for facilities and infrastructure Funding for the development of sustainable activity and education programmes	Public liability laws Local government policies on land use Local government policies on active transport	Perceptions of risks and safety Community attitude towards car-dominated transport, the environment and safety issues
Macro				
Transport	Public transport access and availability	Costs of services and facility provision		
State/federal government	Location of schools and national parks	Contribution to support systems promoting physical education and activity	Policies, standards and guidelines on physical education Policies on land use	Attitudes and beliefs of the department of education towards physical activity and health

Obesogenic elements in microenvironmental settings

Schools

Schools provide an ideal environment to influence the active transport and broader physical activity behaviours of young people. In the past, many school children experienced activity opportunities through physical education (PE). However, recent scholastic pressures have resulted in a reduction in the time allocated to physical education within schools (Jago and Baranowski, 2004). In the United States, it is estimated that primary school children may spend as little as 25 minutes per week performing moderate to vigorous activity in school PE classes (Nader, 2003), while in Europe the duration and intensity of PE programmes appears insufficient to meet current health recommendations (Koutedakis and Bouziotas, 2003). Given that time at school represents approximately 40 per cent of children's waking hours, changes in school policy are required to provide sufficient levels of physical education and sports participation within educational curricula (Fox, 2004). Although there is evidence that children may compensate for reduced activity within school physical education classes by increasing their non-curricular activity (Mallam *et al.*, 2003), many extra-curricular activities, such as active travel to and from school, also require changes to school and government policies (Jago and Baranowski, 2004; Swinburn and Egger, 2002). Such policy emphases should include strategies to facilitate an increase in the number of children who walk and cycle to school and support important adjunct factors such as walking and cycling paths, storage space for bicycles, and well-equipped playground areas. Opportunities for increased physical activity may include during the breaks (recess and lunch), and before and after school (McKenzie *et al.*, 1997; Zask *et al.*, 2001). Strategic use of after school time, however, would necessitate the availability of supervised after-school activity programmes and out-of-hours access to school facilities and equipment, both of which are likely to have an economic impact.

A key sociocultural component of the school as a microenvironment, as it applies to physical activity, is the balance of school time devoted to academic versus active pursuits (Dwyer *et al.*, 2003). The ethos of the school determines the level of support for PE, sport and other physical activity opportunities and the attitudes and beliefs regarding the links between health, fitness, well-being and academic and social achievement (Gittelsohn *et al.*, 2003). Teachers can serve as important role models to children and the potential for this group to prompt physical activity in children should not be overlooked (McKenzie *et al.*, 1997). Rather than considering that physical activity is only possible during PE classes, we need to be more innovative and consider including the possibility of an 'active curriculum', whereby activity is incorporated into the academic curriculum as much as possible. Important enabling factors that would ensure a sustainable programme include adequate training of teachers and the provision of sufficient resources including equipment, plus indoor and outdoor spaces for the conduct of physical activity (Dwyer *et al.*, 2003; Sallis *et al.*, 2001; Thow and Cashel, 2003).

Home

The home environment is another important setting in which physical activity should be fostered as habitual activities within the family. Specifically, the potential role model and influence of parents underpin the participation and beliefs of young people (Swinburn and Egger, 2002). Ideally parents should be models of appropriate behaviour and prominent sources of reinforcement in the lives of their children (Perry *et al.*, 1988; Trost *et al.*, 2001). Parents may be considered the 'gatekeepers', providing opportunities or barriers to facilitate or debilitate their child's participation in physical activity. Thus, Table 11.1 outlines the affinity for car use, parental attitudes, habits and beliefs in relation to physical activity, and parent engagement in physical activity with their children. As role models, parents contribute to the sociocultural component that influences the physical activity of children in the home microenvironment, but simultaneously provide the political element by placing restrictions on the opportunities for physical activity. Like the role of teachers within the school setting, parental support is the main driver of physical activity opportunities in the home setting (Trost *et al.*, 2001). The economic cost of parental time and support, however, must be counterbalanced by family economic factors. Similarly, the provision of sports equipment or activity-promoting toys such as bicycles, and facilities for activity such as sufficient backyard space, while likely to promote physical activity in children, are also dependent on economic factors within the home (McKenzie *et al.*, 1992). Nonetheless, the argument that the cost of activity- and sport-related equipment is a barrier to children's physical activity is offset by the cost implications of purchasing DVD players, TVs and video games associated with promoting sedentary behaviours.

Neighbourhoods

There is a growing body of evidence linking the physical environment of neighbourhoods to commuting practices and physical activity levels of community members. Neighbourhoods that are perceived as aesthetic in nature have generally been shown to promote physical activity and recreational walking among community residents (Duncan and Mummery, 2005; McCormack *et al.*, 2004). In addition, both real and perceived risks, including 'stranger danger,' traffic, animals (a natural hazard) and other children (bullying), have been identified as important barriers to physical activity within children (Bauer, Yang and Austin, 2004; Gielen *et al.*, 2004). Timperio *et al.* (2004) recently reported on associations between perceptions of the local neighbourhood and walking and cycling among 5- to 6- and 10- to 12-year-old Australian children. A major finding was that parental perceptions of the environment were associated with children's walking or cycling behaviours, suggesting that improving road and pedestrian facilities in neighbourhoods and/or perceptions of road safety may be important strategies to increase active transport in youth. In Australia, the provision of off-street recreational and sports facilities such as safe walking and cycle paths, skateboard ramps, and the general attractiveness of open spaces is governed by local governments (Swinburn and Egger, 2002).

In addition to providing off-street recreational areas, local government in-strumentalities have the capacity to influence children's physical activity levels through highly targeted, child-focused education interventions designed to pre-vent pedestrian injuries. Carlin, Taylor and Nolan (1998) argue that bicycle edu-cation courses provide the opportunity to emphasise a safety culture. Participation in bicycle education, along with adequate reinforcement in the home, may help to strike a balance between over-protection and parental restrictions and over-con-fidence, or risk-taking, in young people. Kendrick and Royal (2003) support this contention, reporting that family encouragement was associated with higher rates of helmet wearing among 1,061 year 5 schoolchildren across 28 primary schools in Nottingham, UK. Further, Ehrlich *et al.* (2004) compared parents' and children's attitudes and habits towards use of bicycle helmets and car seatbelts and noted a strong association between parental role models and reduced risk-taking behav-iour by children. These findings underline the need to target parents and families as part of the active commuting and injury intervention process.

Public liability laws, local government policies on active transport and the sup-port of local community members are also important considerations determining physical activity in children within the neighbourhood setting. A major challenge for local governments, particularly in established residential areas, is to ensure an appropriate mix of housing, shops, workplaces and schools within urban environ-ments while maximising the aesthetics and amount of open recreational space. Although both of these factors reportedly influence physical activity levels within communities (Craig *et al.*, 2002; Frank, Andresen and Schmid, 2004), they, in turn, are influenced by commercial pressures arising from macroenvironmental sectors (Frank, 2004).

Macroenvironments

Transport

Numerous aspects of the transport macroenvironment are related to the physi-cal activity levels of children. These include access to and availability of public transport and infrastructure supporting active transport options for walking and cycling. Economic factors of relevance include the costs of services and the provi-sion of facilities. Political decision-making often drives the policies related to fund-ing formulae associated with various transport options. Such political decisions are subsequently influenced by economic forces which are essentially beyond the control of individuals but also govern land-use patterns (Frank, 2004; Swinburn, Egger and Raza, 1999).

Relevant government departments

State government departments with a major role to play in the physical activ-ity participation (and health) of children are education, transport, health, sport and recreation, and families (or the various derivatives). Such departments are also often responsible for the accreditation, training and continuing education of government officers and members of the general public. As for the microenvironments and transport, economic imperatives are driven by policy, cost and political goodwill. From a sociocultural perspective, important issues relevant to all levels of government include the level of engagement and responsibility for the education and health of future generations.

In summary, numerous interrelated micro- and macroenvironments influence the physical activity opportunities of children. Therefore, it is essential that environmental interventions designed to increase the physical activity of children identify and address those contextual influences that are prone to modification. As demonstrated in Table 11.1, the ANGELO grid provides a structured framework that aids in the identification of environmental barriers that reduce physical activity in children. Whereas elements identified within the macroenvironmental sectors tend to be resistant to modification, many elements within the home, school and, to a lesser extent, the neighbourhood setting are relatively ductile and should be addressed by environmental interventions where possible. The balance of this chapter provides a specific example of active commuting (walking to school), and addresses the modifiable barriers to physical activity identified by the ANGELO framework. Despite its relative simplicity, active commuting to and from school represents an important physical activity opportunity with the potential to contribute to the prevention of childhood obesity (Tudor-Locke, Ainsworth and Popkin, 2001). However, in order for active commuting to be a practical and feasible option, and thereby maximise the chance of a positive outcome within a behavioural setting, a concerted effort to identify and address environmental barriers to active transport is required each time the programme is implemented.

Active commuting to school – a sound investment?

In adults, active commuting to work has been shown to result in lowered blood pressure, improved blood lipid profiles, and greater physical fitness (Oja, Vuori and Paronen, 1998; Vuori, Oja and Paronen, 1994). Although controversial (Harten and Olds, 2004; Metcalf *et al.*, 2004; Sleap and Warburton, 1993), it is widely assumed that interventions promoting active transport in children not only produce similar health benefits but also encourage active lifestyle patterns that may be retained in adulthood (Carlin, Taylor and Nolan, 1998). Of particular concern is the suggestion that children who are accustomed to being driven even short distances are not likely to appreciate the benefits of walking as a lifestyle activity when adults (Roberts, 1996a; Sleap and Warburton, 1993). In support of this postulate, empirical evidence suggests that inactive behaviours adopted in childhood track better than active behaviours in the transition from adolescence to young adulthood (Raitakari *et al.*, 1994). Despite these concerns, a consistent message arising from reports worldwide is that fewer children are walking to and from school (Harten and Olds, 2004; Roberts, 1996b; Tudor-Locke, Ainsworth and Popkin, 2001).

To assist in the universal promotion of walking to school, research needs to consider the correlates and antecedents of modes of transport amongst children, parents, communities and schools. Morris and Hardman (1997) have highlighted concerns regarding pedestrian safety amidst traffic, air pollution, and sidewalk and road maintenance. Further, Tudor-Locke, Ainsworth and Popkin (2001) suggest that crime and overall community and school design must be considered along with the parent's real and perceived concerns for their children's safety. Parental concerns regarding the safety of children are not unfounded as pedestrian injuries are a leading cause of death and serious injury for school-aged children (Rivara, 1990), and a large proportion of these injuries occur while children are walking to or from school (Joly, Foggin and Pless, 1991).

Investigations using self-report measures of physical activity have indicated that the exercise behaviour of children is predicated on their enjoyment of physical activity (Stucky-Ropp and DiLorenzo, 1993). A logical extension of this is that poor physical activity experiences may be a significant contributor to reduced levels of physical activity and, consequently, problems in the maintenance of energy balance (Hills and Cambourne, 2002). Thus, wherever possible, physical activity experiences for children must be positive and conducted in a manner that fosters fun and enjoyment. Success in the activity setting is a major determinant of continued participation in activity as success is associated with self-efficacy. Accordingly, youngsters need to experience a measure of success and a sense of belonging in order to maximise habitual physical activity. The goal for each individual should be to participate in physical activity at every opportunity.

Walk-to-School opportunities and programmes are good examples of sustainable environmental strategies to increase physical activity in children (Hills and Cambourne, 2002). Programmes should consist of features to ensure safety whilst meeting the important criteria of being an enjoyable and active learning experience. Walking to school opportunities can create an environment or culture in which children feel comfortable, learning can be fostered and children have fun walking to school (Hills and Cambourne, 2002). A key component of successful programme examples includes sustainability, in which existing community networks and social structures are utilised to positively influence the determinants of physical activity participation. Parental concerns regarding child safety can be addressed by including trained, screened and accredited Walking Leaders and volunteers who take responsibility for the management and supervision of the walking groups in schools. Walking Leaders and volunteers should be equipped with first-aid kits, roll cards, water bottles and emergency telephone numbers, and ideally be identifiable by special uniforms and identification cards. A learning environment can be fostered by engaging staff and volunteers as role models, developing theme days, setting challenges for the children each week and implementing incentive schemes that may include material and non-material items. News regarding active transport can be communicated to students, parents and staff via school newsletters and school assemblies.

Conclusion

In order for a larger number of children to benefit from active commuting to and from school, the use of the ANGELO framework in the context of physical activity reinforces the need for a multi-sectoral approach. Greater collective responsibility needs to be taken by members of the various settings and sectors for viable environmental strategies to increase physical activity and help minimise sedentary behaviours. This approach would undoubtedly also greatly assist in the sustainability of such programmes.

References

Ball, K. and Crawford, D. (2003) 'The obesity epidemic: contextual influences on physical activity and body weight', *Journal of Science and Medicine in Sport*, 6: 377–8.

Bauer, K.W., Yang, Y.W. and Austin, S.B. (2004) '"How can we stay healthy when you're throwing all of this in front of us?" Findings from focus groups and interviews in middle schools on environmental influences on nutrition and physical activity', *Health Education and Behavior*, 31: 34–46.

Burdette, H.L. and Whitaker, R.C. (2004) 'Neighborhood playgrounds, fast food restaurants, and crime: relationships to overweight in low-income preschool children', *Preventive Medicine*, 38: 57–63.

Campbell, K., Waters, E., O'Meara, S., Kelly, S. and Summerbell, C. (2002) 'Interventions for preventing obesity in children', *Cochrane Database of Systematic Reviews*, CD001871.

Carlin, J.B., Taylor, P. and Nolan, T. (1998) 'School based bicycle safety education and bicycle injuries in children: a case-control study', *Injury Prevention*, 4: 22–7.

Craig, C.L., Brownson, R.C., Cragg, S.E. and Dunn, A.L. (2002) 'Exploring the effect of the environment on physical activity: a study examining walking to work', *American Journal of Preventive Medicine*, 23: 36–43.

Crawford, D. and Ball, K. (2002) 'Behavioural determinants of the obesity epidemic', *Asia Pacific Journal of Clinical Nutrition*, 11: S718–21.

Duncan, M. and Mummery, K. (2005) 'Psychosocial and environmental factors associated with physical activity among city dwellers in regional Queensland', *Preventive Medicine*, 40: 363–72.

Dwyer, J.J., Allison, K.R., Barrera, M., Hansen, B., Goldenberg, E. and Boutilier, M.A. (2003) 'Teachers' perspective on barriers to implementing physical activity curriculum guidelines for school children in Toronto', *Canadian Journal of Public Health*, 94: 448–52.

Egger, G. and Swinburn, B. (1997) 'An "ecological" approach to the obesity pandemic', *British Medical Journal*, 315: 477–81.

Ehrlich, P.F., Helmkamp, J.C., Williams, J.M., Haque, A. and Furbee, P.M. (2004) 'Matched analysis of parent's and children's attitudes and practices towards motor vehicle and bicycle safety: an important information gap', *Injury Control and Safety Promotion*, 11: 23–8.

Fox, K.R. (2004) 'Childhood obesity and the role of physical activity', *Journal of the Royal Society of Health*, 124: 34–9.

Frank, L.D. (2004) 'Economic determinants of urban form: resulting trade-offs between active and sedentary forms of travel', *American Journal of Preventive Medicine*, 27: 146–53.

Frank, L.D., Andresen, M.A. and Schmid, T.L. (2004) 'Obesity relationships with community design, physical activity, and time spent in cars', *American Journal of Preventive Medicine*, 27: 87–96.

Garcia, A.W., Broda, M.A., Frenn, M., Coviak, C., Pender, N.J. and Ronis, D.L. (1995) 'Gender and developmental differences in exercise beliefs among youth and prediction of their exercise behavior', *Journal of School Health*, 65: 213–19.

Gielen, A.C., Defrancesco, S., Bishai, D., Mahoney, P., Ho, S. and Guyer, B. (2004) 'Child pedestrians: the role of parental beliefs and practices in promoting safe walking in urban neighborhoods', *Journal of Urban Health*, 81: 545–55.

Gittelsohn, J., Merkle, S., Story, M., Stone, E.J., Steckler, A., Noel, J., Davis, S., Martin, C.J. and Ethelbah, B. (2003) 'School climate and implementation of the Pathways study', *Preventive Medicine*, 37: S97–106.

Harten, N. and Olds, T. (2004) 'Patterns of active transport in 11–12 year old Australian children', *Australian and New Zealand Journal of Public Health*, 28: 167–72.

Hills, A.P. and Cambourne, B. (2002) 'Walking to school – a sustainable environmental strategy to prevent childhood obesity', *Australian Epidemiologist*, 9: 15–18.

Jago, R. and Baranowski, T. (2004) 'Non-curricular approaches for increasing physical activity in youth: a review', *Preventive Medicine*, 39: 157–63.

Jequier, E. (2002) 'Pathways to obesity', *International Journal of Obesity and Related Metabolic Disorders*, 26: S12–17.

Jequier, E. and Tappy, L. (1999) 'Regulation of body weight in humans', *Physiological Reviews*, 79: 451–80.

Joly, M.F., Foggin, P.M. and Pless, I.B. (1991) 'Geographical and socio-ecological variations of traffic accidents among children', *Social Science and Medicine*, 33: 765–9.

Kendrick, D. and Royal, S. (2003) 'Inequalities in cycle helmet use: cross sectional survey in schools in deprived areas of Nottingham', *Archives of Disease in Childhood*, 88: 876–80.

Koutedakis, Y. and Bouziotas, C. (2003) 'National physical education curriculum: motor and cardiovascular health related fitness in Greek adolescents', *British Journal of Sports Medicine*, 37: 311–14.

Loke, K.Y. (2002) 'Consequences of childhood and adolescent obesity', *Asia Pacific Journal of Clinical Nutrition*, 11: S702–4.

McCormack, G., Giles-Corti, B., Lange, A., Smith, T., Martin, K. and Pikora, T.J. (2004) 'An update of recent evidence of the relationship between objective and self-report measures of the physical environment and physical activity behaviours', *Journal of Science and Medicine in Sport*, 7: 81–92.

McGuire, M.T., Wing, R.R., Klem, M.L. and Hill, J.O. (1999) 'Behavioral strategies of individuals who have maintained long-term weight losses', *Obesity Reviews*, 7: 334–41.

McKenzie, T.L., Sallis, J.F., Elder, J.P., Berry, C.C., Hoy, P.L., Nader, P.R., Zive, M.M. and Broyles, S.L. (1997) 'Physical activity levels and prompts in young children at recess: a two-year study of a bi-ethnic sample', *Research Quarterly for Exercise and Sport*, 68: 195–202.

McKenzie, T.L., Sallis, J.F., Nader, P.R., Broyles, S.L. and Nelson, J.A. (1992) 'Anglo- and Mexican-American preschoolers at home and at recess: activity patterns and environmental influences', *Journal of Developmental and Behavioral Pediatrics*, 13: 173–80.

Maddock, J. (2004) 'The relationship between obesity and the prevalence of fast food restaurants: state-level analysis', *American Journal of Health Promotion*, 19: 137–43.

Mallam, K.M., Metcalf, B.S., Kirkby, J., Voss, L.D. and Wilkin, T.J. (2003) 'Contribution of timetabled physical education to total physical activity in primary school children: cross sectional study', *British Medical Journal*, 327: 592–3.

Marti, A., Moreno-Aliaga, M.J., Hebebrand, J. and Martinez, J.A. (2004) 'Genes, life-styles and obesity', *International Journal of Obesity and Related Metabolic Disorders*, 28: S29–36.

Metcalf, B., Voss, L., Jeffery, A., Perkins, J. and Wilkin, T. (2004) 'Physical activity cost of the school run: impact on schoolchildren of being driven to school', *British Medical Journal*, 329: 832–83.

Morris, J.N. and Hardman, A.E. (1997) 'Walking to health', *Sports Medicine*, 23: 306–32.

Nader, P.R. (2003) 'Frequency and intensity of activity of third-grade children in physical education', *Archives of Pediatrics and Adolescent Medicine*, 157: 185–90.

Ochoa, M.C., Marti, A., Azcona, C., Chueca, M., Oyarzabal, M., Pelach, R., Patino, A., Moreno-Aliaga, M.J., Martinez-Gonzalez, M.A. and Martinez, J.A. (2004) 'Gene–gene interaction between PPARgamma2 and ADRbeta3 increases obesity risk in children and adolescents', *International Journal of Obesity and Related Metabolic Disorders*, 28: S37–41.

Oja, P., Vuori, I. and Paronen, O. (1998) 'Daily walking and cycling to work: their utility as health-enhancing physical activity', *Patient Education and Counseling*, 33: S87–94.

Perry, C.L., Luepker, R.V., Murray, D.M., Kurth, C., Mullis, R., Crockett, S. and Jacobs, D.R., Jr (1988) 'Parent involvement with children's health promotion: the Minnesota Home Team', *American Journal of Public Health*, 78: 1156–60.

Raitakari, O.T., Porkka, K.V., Taimela, S., Telama, R., Räsänen, L. and Viikari, J.S. (1994) 'Effects of persistent physical activity and inactivity on coronary risk factors in children and young adults: the Cardiovascular Risk in Young Finns Study', *American Journal of Epidemiology*, 140: 195–205.

Rivara, F.P. (1990) 'Child pedestrian injuries in the United States: current status of the problem, potential interventions, and future research needs', *American Journal of Diseases of Children*, 144: 692–6.

Roberts, I. (1996a) 'Children and sport: walking to school has future benefits', *British Medical Journal*, 312: 1229.

Roberts, I. (1996b) 'Safely to school?' *Lancet*, 347: 1642.

Sallis, J.F., Conway, T.L., Prochaska, J.J., McKenzie, T.L., Marshall, S.J. and Brown, M. (2001) 'The association of school environments with youth physical activity', *American Journal of Public Health*, 91: 618–20.

Sleap, M. and Warburton, P. (1993) 'Are primary school children gaining heart health benefits from their journeys to school?' *Child: Care, Health and Development*, 19: 99–108.

Stucky-Ropp, R.C. and DiLorenzo, T.M. (1993) 'Determinants of exercise in children', *Preventive Medicine*, 22: 880–9.

Swinburn, B. and Egger, G. (2002) 'Preventive strategies against weight gain and obesity', *Obesity Reviews*, 3: 289–301.

Swinburn, B., Egger, G. and Raza, F. (1999) 'Dissecting obesogenic environments: the development and application of a framework for identifying and prioritizing environmental interventions for obesity', *Preventive Medicine*, 29: 563–70.

Thow, A.M. and Cashel, K.M. (2003) 'Nutrition and physical activity interventions in the school – is it a win–win situation?' *Asia Pacific Journal of Clinical Nutrition*, 12: S16.

Timperio, A., Crawford, D., Telford, A. and Salmon, J. (2004) 'Perceptions about the local neighborhood and walking and cycling among children', *Preventive Medicine*, 38: 39–47.

Trost, S.G., Kerr, L.M., Ward, D.S. and Pate, R.R. (2001) 'Physical activity and determinants of physical activity in obese and non-obese children', *International Journal of Obesity and Related Metabolic Disorders*, 25: 822–9.

Tudor-Locke, C., Ainsworth, B.E. and Popkin, B.M. (2001) 'Active commuting to school: an overlooked source of children's physical activity?', *Sports Medicine*, 31: 309–13.

Vuori, I.M., Oja, P. and Paronen, O. (1994) 'Physically active commuting to work – testing its potential for exercise promotion', *Medicine and Science in Sports and Exercise*, 26: 844–50.

Zask, A., van Beurden, E., Barnett, L., Brooks, L.O. and Dietrich, U.C. (2001) 'Active school playgrounds – myth or reality? Results of the "move it groove it" project', *Preventive Medicine*, 33: 402–8.

12 Interventions for the prevention and management of childhood obesity

B. Deforche, I. De Bourdeaudhuij and A.P. Hills

Introduction

Prevention of childhood obesity

Energy balance occurs when energy intake (food intake) equals energy expenditure. Energy intake in excess of energy expenditure results in weight gain. Total energy expenditure consists of three components: resting metabolic rate (60–70 per cent), the thermic effect of food (15–20 per cent) and the energy expended in physical activity (20–25 per cent). Physical activity is the component most susceptible to change. Therefore, interventions aimed at preventing childhood obesity should focus on factors that influence food intake and physical activity.

Prevention of obesity should commence very early in life. For example, breast-feeding an infant is preferable to the use of a formula and may contribute to the prevention of obesity (Dietz, 2001). Further, young children's food and activity choices can be influenced by early intervention and guidance (Birch and Fisher, 1998) and habits learned early in life are likely to carry through to adulthood (Kelder *et al.*, 1994).

Educating the families of young children concerning nutrition and physical activity may have a powerful positive impact on the obesity risk of children, especially those with obese parents. Obesity prevention programmes should target the whole population, as it is difficult to identify children at risk of developing obesity at a very young age (Power, Lake and Cole, 1997). Risk factors for developing obesity include genetic, social and behavioural factors. Since genetic and social factors cannot be changed, prevention programmes have to focus on behavioural changes including increasing physical activity and reducing energy intake. When focusing on healthy eating (rather than reducing energy intake) and enjoyable physical activities, all children at risk or not at risk of developing obesity may benefit from an intervention programme. Such an approach should also minimise any associated risk of negatively influencing behaviour and predisposing eating disorders.

Interventions within the family

Family lifestyles play a central role in the development of children's food preferences and activity choices. Parents in particular have a strong influence on their children's lifestyles through modelling and education (Hodges, 2003). Therefore it is vital that strategies aimed at preventing childhood obesity involve parents and the wider family unit. A competing challenge however to changing family nutritional and activity habits is the knowledge that they result from interplay of deep-rooted sociocultural, ethnic and environmental factors.

Parental influences are early determinants of food attitudes and practices in young children (Birch and Davison, 2001) and parenting styles may influence the development of food preferences and the ability of the child to regulate intake. Efforts by parents to control the food intake of children can interfere with children's ability to regulate their own food intake (Birch and Fisher, 1998). Therefore, although parents should be in charge of what children are offered and when and where it is offered, children should be allowed to choose from the foods offered and control how much they eat (Evers, 1997). Box 12.1 provides some general nutritional guidelines for parents to help in the prevention of obesity in young children.

Box 12.1 Nutritional guidelines to prevent obesity in young children

Prepare a variety of foods (with servings from all five groups: grains and cereals, meat and protein, fruit and vegetables, dairy, fats)

Eat home-prepared meals as often as possible

Provide plenty of fruits, vegetables and food rich in starch and fibre (wholemeal bread, pasta, rice or cereals instead of white equivalents)

Avoid consumption of high-fat foods (choose semi-skimmed milk, low-fat margarines, spreads and yoghurts)

Reduce the use of fat during food preparation (grill, boil or steam foods rather than frying)

Minimise the use of high-sugar foods. For example, avoid adding sugar to cereals and drinks

Limit consumption of sugar-sweetened soft drinks; as an alternative encourage drinking water

Encourage the consumption of food and drink in the kitchen or at the dining table

Avoid eating at times other than mealtimes and recognised snack periods

Eat family meals together whenever possible

Serve appropriate portion sizes

Encourage children to eat a healthy breakfast and avoid skipping meals

Minimise unhealthy snacking (for example, high in sugar and/or fat), especially after dinnertime

Make healthy snacks (fruits, carrots and other vegetables) attractive and readily available

Provide a healthy lunch box to take to school

Teach children that it is okay to leave food on their plate when they have had sufficient

Do not use food as a reward

Parents have the responsibility to make healthy choices while shopping, to prepare healthy low-fat meals and to make healthy snacks (such as fruits) readily available to children. Parents should also take special care to have meals at regular times with the whole family whenever possible, to be realistic with portion sizes and to limit eating to one place, such as the kitchen or dining table with no eating in front of the television. Most importantly, children should never skip meals or be forced to finish the entire meal. Rather, children should be taught to respond to body signals of hunger and fullness (Rolland-Cachera and Bellisle, 2002) in order to self-regulate energy intake better and not overeat. The use of food as a reward or to regulate mood and behaviour is totally inappropriate (Rolland-Cachera and Bellisle, 2002).

Parental support and modelling are strong determinants of children's physical activity level (Fogelholm *et al.*, 1999). When parents are engaged in physical activities and sports, their children are more likely to have a positive attitude towards physical activity. In contrast, parents who habitually watch television for extended periods of time will promote sedentary attitudes and behaviours in their children. Parental support may be in the form of transport to playgrounds or sport facilities, enrolment in sports clubs, buying basic sports equipment, reminding children to be active, being active together with their children and encouraging active play outside. Ideally, parents should expose children to as many different kinds of physical activities as possible. This should include sports participation and the implementation of lifestyle activities as part of their children's daily routine. Parents should encourage children to take the stairs rather than the elevator, to walk the dog, to walk or cycle to and from school or the shop, and to do household activities (such as doing the dishes, cleaning their room, washing the car, gardening etc.). Unfortunately, such lifestyle activities have reduced substantially in the past 50 years as industrialisation and automation of society has advanced.

Another strategy to increase physical activity in children is to limit television viewing time. When children are encouraged to reduce their television viewing time, their attitudes towards vigorous physical activity are more positive than when they are encouraged to increase their physical activity (Epstein *et al.*, 1995a). That is, when children are urged to increase their physical activity levels, they perceive the encouragement as a forced choice. In contrast, the encouragement to reduce television time provides the young person with the chance to choose a substitute. Unfortunately, television viewing promotes both reduced activity and increased food consumption. Many children snack while watching television; in addition, children's food choices are easily influenced by television advertisements such as for soft drinks and energy-dense foods (Kraak and Pelletier, 1998).

Reductions in television viewing time have the potential to decrease the consumption of energy-dense foods and also to increase the likelihood that time will be spent in more energy-intensive activities. Parents should be careful that television viewing does not become integrated into the daily routine of their children. For example, if the television is used as a babysitter when children are small this may become a habit that is difficult to alter later. Box 12.2 provides some physical activity guidelines for parents to use in the prevention of obesity in young children.

> *Box 12.2* Physical activity guidelines to prevent obesity in young children
>
> Provide opportunities for safe active play both inside and outside the home
> Expose children to as many different kinds of physical activity as possible
> Enrol children in sports clubs
> Organise physical activities with the entire family at least once a week
> Encourage walking or cycling to and from school or the shop
> Encourage taking the stairs rather than the elevator. If there are too many floors, encourage walking some of the flights and try to increase gradually the number of flights walked
> Involve the children in home activities such as doing the dishes, cleaning their room, washing the car, gardening, walking the dog etc.
> Limit time watching television or playing computer games to less than two hours per day
> Only allow children to watch television if they have been physically active for at least one hour
> Do not allow televisions and computer games in children's bedrooms

School-based interventions

Schools are an ideal setting for the prevention of childhood obesity. School programmes offer many advantages including large numbers of children to be reached, guidance can be continuous, costs can be minimised and parents can be easily involved in the programme. No other public institution has as much contact with children and their parents as the school. Parents can be involved through meetings and educational material can be sent to the family home. Schools have the potential and the personnel to promote changes in physical activity and eating behaviour. Schools need not only to teach healthy living in classroom health education but also to implement healthy living.

Physical education classes provide a unique opportunity to contribute to increased physical activity levels in children. There is also great potential to utilise break times better, including before, during and after school for physical activity and sports. Most schools have a range of sport facilities and equipment and generally these are only used minimally after school hours. It is also logical for schools to promote active transport to and from school. The school environment also provides great potential for multiple food and nutrition activities, experiences and exposures. Examples include food that is available at school, in vending machines, at fundraising events and parties, and as classroom snacks. Nutrition interventions at school should help students make healthy food choices by preparing healthy school lunches (low in fat and rich in fresh fruit and vegetables) and providing healthy alternatives to soft drinks and sweets such as fruits and cold water through dispensers. Teacher training is also needed to foster knowledge and understanding of key physical activity and eating concepts and behaviour change strategies (see below). Physical education teachers could act as coordinators of school-based intervention programmes for the prevention of obesity. In addition, other school or community staff such as a nurse or doctor could screen children for overweight. Children identified as overweight could be referred to a clinic-based weight management programme to prevent further weight gain. To date, a number of effective school-based interventions have been reported (Story, 1999); however, they have limited potential for more widespread implementation. Box 12.3 provides some suggested guidelines for the development of a school-based obesity prevention programme.

Interventions within the community

Governments need to financially and physically support obesity prevention programmes. In terms of supporting healthy eating, governments should take action to make healthy food (such as fresh fruits and vegetables) easily available to those who perceive healthy food as expensive or difficult to obtain. Governments can legislate on food labelling, food advertisements directed at children, and school food policies. In terms of supporting physical activity, they should take responsibility to provide, for example, safe environments and roads that encourage walking and cycling, and areas and facilities for active play and sports. They should give prominence to staircases rather than elevators in public buildings. They could also expand the physical activity and health education component of school curricula, as well as provide information and guidelines for healthy living including the importance of healthy eating and regular physical activity.

Treatment of childhood obesity

Aim of treatment

Prevention is recognised as the primary and most efficient means to combat obesity; however, many children and adolescents who are already overweight or obese require assistance to prevent further weight gain and to prevent development of

---

Box 12.3 Guidelines to develop a school-based obesity prevention programme

Provide classroom health education related to healthy nutrition and physical activity
Involve parents through meetings and educational material sent to the home
Provide physical education classes that total at least two hours per week
Provide active opportunities at break times before, during and after school
Provide a variety of sports and lifestyle activities
Promote active transport to and from school
Prepare healthy school lunches (low in fat and rich in fresh vegetables and fruits)
Encourage the consumption of healthy alternatives such as cold water and fruits instead of soft drinks and sweets
Provide teacher training on the key physical activity and eating concepts and behaviour change strategies
Refer overweight children to a clinic-based weight management programme

obesity-related co-morbidities in adulthood. Treatment should start as early as possible. The earlier treatment starts, the greater the chance of long-term success (Epstein *et al.*, 1995b). Frequently, there is a incorrect belief that the child will outgrow the problem. Early identification and management of children who exceed a healthy weight for height, gender and age will prevent the increasing incidence of paediatric obesity and will decrease the potential for associated medical and psycho-social problems in adulthood. The aim of childhood obesity treatment is gradual and controlled weight loss allowing for normal growth and development and causing minimal hunger (Schonfeld-Warden and Warden, 1997). The treatment goal depends on the age of the child and the severity of the weight problem. In young children who have mild to moderate weight problems, weight maintenance or reduced rates of weight gain may be sufficient because future growth will normalise body weight. Among severely obese children and adolescents, the treatment goal is weight reduction at a rate of 0.5–1.0 kg/month (Schonfeld-Warden and Warden, 1997). Because children normally gain approximately 5 kg per year, the effect of a 5 kg weight loss is doubled (Dietz, 1999). Too often, children and their parents have unrealistic expectations about the magnitude and rate of weight loss. Weight loss is likely to be more sustainable if achieved slowly, since gradual changes in overweight are more likely to be due to loss of fat mass than loss of fat-free mass. The goal of all weight control programmes should be reduction in excess fat. Even modest reductions in excess fat can reduce health risks (Epstein *et al.*, 1989; Pidlich *et al.*, 1997). In growing children, fat loss can be compatible with no loss of weight or even slight weight gain. Thus, success of treatment should be evaluated as either the attainment of a body of normal fatness or achieving sufficient reduction in body mass to enhance health and physical fitness. Achieving ideal weight for height, age and gender should be considered an unrealistic goal.

Obesity results from an energy intake in excess of energy expenditure. A relatively small imbalance between energy input and expenditure can lead to significant weight gain over time. Most children demonstrate a small but consistent weight gain over several years (Dietz, Bandini and Gortmaker, 1990). The basis of weight reduction is to alter the energy balance so that energy expenditure exceeds energy intake. For successful weight reduction, negative energy balance must continue for a significant period of time, in many cases for months or years. Weight loss can be induced by a reduction in energy consumed (food intake), an increase in energy expended in physical activity or a combination of both. Therefore, treatment programmes could focus on modifying eating and/or physical activity behaviours of the obese child. Eating and physical activity patterns are learned behaviours and can be modified. The multidisciplinary approach of a comprehensive behavioural lifestyle programme including changes in physical activity and eating practices has been identified as the most effective strategy in weight management in children and adolescents (Fulton *et al.*, 2001). A family approach in which parents learn to support their child is an essential component of successful weight management (Epstein, 1996). Whereas the basic treatment principles are valid for all children and adolescents, several individual factors have to be taken into account, for example age, degree of overweight, parental obesity and social aspects.

Treatment components

Nutrition

The basis for nutritional modification in obesity treatment is the hypothesis that obese individuals consume too much energy in relation to their energy expenditure. The purpose is to reduce caloric intake below the child's energy expenditure. Because children are continuing to grow and develop, the diet should be well balanced, providing sufficient calories and all essential nutrients for growth (Robinson, 1999). The focus should be on healthy eating rather than slimming. It is better to avoid using the word 'diet' when talking to the children. For many children the word 'diet' conveys messages of deprivation, avoidance of favourite foods and the need to eat small portions of foods they do not enjoy (Barker and Cooke, 1992). Furthermore, 'diet' is often considered to be something that needs to be followed only until the desired weight loss has been achieved, after which it can be abandoned and the unhealthy eating habits which contributed to the excess weight can be resumed (Grace, 2001). Weight control will require lifelong attention; therefore food should be tasty and nutritional changes should be acceptable to the children and their parents in the long term. Many overweight and obese children perceive high-fat snack foods such as chocolate and biscuits to be 'forbidden' foods. Banning foods and striving for the perfect diet can be counterproductive (Grace, 2001). It tends to lead to increased cravings for such foods and preoccupation with food and appearance, which may predispose them to eating disorders in the future. Chocolates and biscuits can be part of a healthy diet as long as the amounts and the frequency of consumption are limited. Dietary restrictions should not be presented in a punitive manner. Focus should rather be on all the different foods they are allowed to eat. The dietary changes should be simple and unambiguous, so that it is easy to implement for the children. Box 12.4 summarises guidelines for nutritional intervention in obese children.

Dependent on the degree of obesity and age of the child, different dietary

---

Box 12.4 Guidelines for nutritional intervention in obese children

Provide sufficient calories and all essential nutrients for growth
Focus on healthy eating rather than slimming
Food should be tasty and dietary changes should be acceptable to the children in the long term
Focus on all the different foods they are allowed to eat, rather than on what foods are being restricted
High-fat foods such as chocolates and biscuits can be part of a healthy diet as long as the amounts and the frequency of consumption are limited
Dietary changes should be easy to implement for the children
In young and overweight children nutritional counselling may be sufficient
Balanced low-calorie diets may be appropriate for moderately obese children
Very low-calorie diets should be limited to morbidly obese children and should only be used during a limited period of time and under close medical supervision

interventions are necessary (Zwiauer, 2000). In young and overweight children nutritional counselling (as described under obesity prevention) may be sufficient. In moderately obese children some caloric restriction may be required. Severe caloric restriction should be limited to morbidly obese children and applied under strict medical supervision.

Balanced low-calorie diet

In balanced low-calorie diets, the energy intake is reduced by about one-third (Caroli and Burniat, 2002). Nutrient content remains balanced with 20 per cent of energy derived from protein, 30–35 per cent from fat and 45–50 per cent from carbohydrate. Generally, these diets do not need supplementation with minerals and vitamins. Usually a fixed number of meals are recommended (mostly five meals per day) in order to avoid snacking or skipping meals. It is also important to recommend sufficient fluid intake (1.5–2 L/day), preferably water. With balanced low-calorie diets, weight loss of approximately 0.5 kg/week can be achieved even over longer periods (Zwiauer, 2000).

Epstein and Squires (1988) have developed the Traffic Light Diet, which is an approach to make balanced low-calorie diets easily understandable and more attractive to children. The Traffic Light Diet divides food into five categories: fruits and vegetables; grain; milk and dairy; protein; and other. Each category is subdivided by calorie content into the three colours of the traffic light: red (stop), yellow (proceed with caution) and green (go). Red foods are those that are high in fat or simple carbohydrate calories and low in nutrient density. Yellow foods are the staples of the diet that supply basic nutrition. Green foods are low in fat and high in nutrient density, and presented only in the fruit and vegetable and other groups. Each category of food includes both yellow and red foods, and in many instances a yellow food becomes a red food by the manner of preparation (frying versus steaming etc.). Children count the number of servings consumed for each traffic light colour. The major goal is to provide the most nutrition for the lowest caloric cost. The diet maximises choice of healthy foods based on individual and familial preferences. The emphasis is on all the different foods they are allowed to eat, rather than on what foods are being restricted. Such an explicit diet classification makes goal-setting, monitoring and feedback possible.

Very low-calorie diet

Very low-calorie diets (VLCDs) should be limited to morbidly obese children for whom rapid weight reduction is essential, and should only be used under close medical supervision (Widhalm and Zwiauer, 1987). These diets usually provide 800 kcal/day or fewer (Caroli and Burniat, 2002). The protein-sparing modified fast (PSMF) is the most commonly used VLCD in the treatment of childhood obesity. It is an unbalanced diet (protein 66 per cent, fat 24 per cent, carbohydrate 10 per cent) and is supposed to spare fat-free mass while producing rapid weight loss (Caroli and Burniat, 2002). Usually, vitamin and mineral supplements are prescribed. Most diets are composed of normal, natural protein-rich foods, but they can also be prepared as special liquid formulas. These VLCDs should be used only for a limited period of time (Zwiauer, 2000). They are useful only during the initial period of treatment and do not lead to long-term changes of lifestyle, which are necessary for weight stabilisation. Following a VLCD, children should gradually increase energy intake by progressing to a balanced low-calorie diet and eventually to a balanced normal-calorie diet.

Negative consequences of dietary interventions

A major concern about the effects of dieting on obese children is the loss of fat-free mass, particularly when the diet is very low in energy (Caroli and Burniat, 2002). A loss of fat-free mass of no more than 25 per cent of total weight loss is considered within the safe range (Stallings *et al.*, 1988), since obesity is associated with increased fat-free mass for height, age and gender. As fat-free mass is a site of high energy expenditure, reduced fat-free mass often results in a decrease in basal metabolic rate, making it harder to lose weight or increasing the risk of weight regain (Maffeis, Schutz and Pinelli, 1992). Another potential negative effect of dietary interventions in children is reduced growth velocity (Amador *et al.*, 1990). Close medical supervision of growth data in children undergoing dietary restrictions must be guaranteed.

Exercise and physical activity

Weight loss is easier to achieve with caloric restrictions than with increases in energy expenditure (Ballor and Keesey, 1991). Although weight loss directly attributable to increased physical activity may be small, physical activity should be an essential part of any weight management programme. Some of the negative side effects of dietary restriction can be avoided by increasing physical activity. Physical activity may preserve or even increase fat-free mass during weight reduction (Sothern *et al.*, 1999). This is important in the long term as fat-free mass largely determines resting metabolic rate, the degree of energy expended in rest, which is the greatest part of total energy expenditure. Therefore, effective weight loss is most likely to occur when a combination of diet and exercise is recommended. Physical activity further enhances negative energy balance. The more calories are expended through physical activity, the less severe dietary restriction is needed. In addition, participation in physical activity may improve psychological well-being and cardiovascular fitness (Grilo, 1994; Treuth *et al.*, 1998). Most importantly, physical activity plays an important role in the maintenance of weight loss (Tremblay, Doucet and Imbeault, 1999).

Motivating obese subjects to adhere to an activity programme is a major challenge. To encourage adherence to physical activity in obese children and adolescents, one must develop an exercise programme that is manageable for them. Interventions that are not tailored to the capabilities of obese participants may

Box 12.5 Guidelines to develop an exercise programme for obese children

Choose aerobic activities
Limit weight-bearing activities at the start of the intervention
Include resistance training
Incorporate postural, flexibility, coordination and breathing exercises
Develop basic movement skills
Choose music that is appropriate for the speed of movements to be performed to motivate the children
Choose games and fun activities
Choose activities which are tailored to the capabilities of the children
Give the children the opportunity to choose activities they like
Increase amount and intensity of activities gradually
Initially the emphasis should be placed on the duration of the exercise rather than on intensity
Make sure children have an opportunity to drink water before, during and after exercise
Provide warm-up and cooling-down periods
Encourage 60 minutes of moderate- to high-intensity activity per day
Organise separate exercise sessions for obese children
Combine a structured exercise programme with the promotion of lifestyle activities

contribute to discouragement of future participation in physical activity. Box 12.5 summarises guidelines to develop an exercise programme for obese children.

Programmed exercise

The major aim of including physical activity in a weight reduction programme is increasing energy expenditure and reducing excess fat. This is best achieved by sustained aerobic exercises that use large muscle groups (trunk, thighs, shoulders). Therefore aerobic exercise such as brisk walking, swimming, cycling, rollerblading and dancing is the most suitable form of exercise for weight reduction. Aquatic activities are physiologically and motivationally optimal activities for obese children. Obese individuals float better in water and tolerate the cool water better than lean people. In water there is a better conduction of body heat, which is sometimes a problem in obese children because of the large amount of subcutaneous fat. Additionally, it is difficult to overload the articular system as a function of excess weight in water. Most obese children like aquatic activities because they are less exhausting and their body is submerged under water. Unfortunately, most of them are embarrassed to be seen in a bathing suit. In severely obese children, weight-bearing activities, such as running or rope skipping, should be limited at the start of an intervention. Activities of this type may discourage the continued participation because of the great energy cost to move their body but, most importantly, moving or lifting the excess body weight may overload their joints. A progressive introduction of weight-bearing aerobic activities is recommended in these children. Enjoyable non-weight-bearing alternatives such as cycling, swimming or other aquatic activities should be the focus in the early stages of a weight reduction programme in severely obese children. The first goal should be to decrease fat levels as this will automatically provide health and fitness benefits. Once fitness levels have improved or fatness levels have decreased, weight-bearing tasks may be much less exhausting and can be progressively implemented into the programme.

In addition to aerobic activities, it is important to incorporate resistance training into the exercise programme. Resistance training is especially important to preserve fat-free mass in children under severe caloric restriction. Sustained resistance training may prevent weight regain after successful treatment. As most obese children have considerable muscular strength, they perform very well on resistance exercises. Exercises aimed at correcting posture and breathing should be an important component of the exercise therapy for obese children. The exercise programme should develop speed, flexibility, coordination, endurance, strength, agility and general fitness. It is important that obese children master some basic movement skills that enable them to participate later in sports and activities together with non-obese peers. Exercise programmes should be preceded and followed by gradual warm-up and cooling-down periods. Children should get the opportunity to drink water before, during and after exercise.

The total amount (duration, frequency) and intensity of activities should be increased gradually to avoid possible discouragement and overload. An understanding of exercise prescription and progression based on intensity and duration of exercise is critical. Initially, the intensity of exercise should be low to moderate to allow sustained duration of exercises adequate to promote a significant fat oxidation. For the first 20 to 30 minutes of exercise, carbohydrate is the predominant fuel; as exercise duration increases beyond 30 minutes, there is an increased reliance on fat stores for energy. At low to moderate intensities (50–70 per cent of the maximal heart rate) fat is the predominant fuel; at high intensities (higher than 70 per cent) there is a greater reliance on carbohydrate for energy. Activities of moderate intensity (such as brisk walking) are less exhausting than high intensity activities (such as running) and therefore more enjoyable and more easily sustained. In the beginning, the intensity of the activity should allow children to talk when performing the activity or children should report a rating of 9–13 on the Borg scale. If body signals such as excessive sweating or breathing, joint pain, dizziness or stitches appear, decrease the exercise intensity and progress more slowly. Having fostered and encouraged enjoyment in physical activity, the intensity of the programme could be increased to allow improvement of aerobic fitness. Improved fitness is accompanied with a decrease in obesity-related health risks (Blair and Brodney, 1999). The total amount of physical activity should eventually be 60 minutes of moderate- to high-intensity activity daily, according to the current recommended frequency of exercise in children (Biddle, Cavill and Sallis, 1998). Of course this should also be increased gradually. To prevent weight gain after successful weight reduction, the recommended amount of physical activity is even higher (Saris *et al.*, 2003).

Since obese children are often embarrassed to be physically active with non-obese peers, it is recommended to organise separate exercise sessions in an initial treatment phase. The activities should be fun and enjoyable for all for them to continue. The enjoyment children gain from physical participation depends to a large extent on their perception of ability or self-mastery (Craig, Goldberg and Dietz, 1996). Always choose activities that are tailored to the capabilities of the obese child and have a high probability of success. The generally low level of self-efficacy in obese children and the need to improve self-esteem makes success in any activity an important motivating factor. Generally, obese children enjoy participating in dancing activities or listening to music while exercising. Choose music that is appropriate for the speed of movements to be performed and that will motivate the children. Another way to motivate children is to let them choose the kinds of activity they want to pursue from a list of activities. Providing a choice of activities appears to be superior to providing a specific exercise prescription in obese children (Epstein *et al.*, 1982). Children may be more likely to continue being active over time, if they have the opportunity to choose their own activities.

Lifestyle activities

Lifestyle programmes attempt not only to increase caloric expenditure, but also to implement physical activities into daily lifestyle. Lifestyle programmes provide the opportunity to divide the caloric expenditure into several small bouts rather than requiring the exercise to be performed in one bout as in a structured exercise programme. Lifestyle activities which can be easily implemented into daily routine include walking or cycling to and from school, active recess, walking the dog, talking the stairs instead of the elevator, gardening and other household activities. According to Epstein *et al.* (1982) changes in lifestyle activities are more effective in maintaining long-term weight loss in obese children than structured exercise. Lifestyle activities are more easily implemented into daily routines and are usually of lower intensity than activities performed in a structured exercise programme. Even light activity can provide a valuable addition to energy expenditure. However, activities of low intensity will not be sufficient to prevent weight regain after successful weight reduction. In particular, activities of moderate to high intensity contribute to weight maintenance after treatment (Jakicic, 2002). Thus, a structured exercise programme that gradually increases the duration and intensity of activities in combination with promoting lifestyle activities may be the most suitable exercise programme for obese children.

Decreasing sedentary activities

In addition to increasing activity levels, it is also important to encourage children to decrease participation in sedentary activities such as television viewing, playing computer games or surfing on the Internet. Epstein *et al.* (1991) demonstrated that obese children often choose to be sedentary rather than active. Reducing sedentary behaviours may be even more effective than promoting physical activity itself for increasing activity levels in obese children. Removing television and computer games will stimulate the child to find substitutes for these sedentary behaviours. If the environment provides easy access to active rather than sedentary alternatives, active behaviours may be chosen. It is however possible that, when the most preferred sedentary behaviours are made less accessible, other sedentary behaviours will be chosen instead of active behaviours. Therefore a combination of discouraging sedentary activities and promoting physical activities may be needed.

Family involvement

Direct involvement of one parent as an active participant in the weight-loss process or modifying parental behaviour is important in weight regulation in obese children (McLean *et al.*, 2003). This is not surprising since parents have a significant impact on the health behaviour and education of their children. It has been demonstrated that the long-term effectiveness of a weight control programme is significantly improved when the intervention is directed at the parents as well as the child, rather than aimed at the child alone (Epstein, 1996). Assessment of the family's readiness to change represents the first focus of therapy. Parents need to learn how to support their children in achieving the desired behavioural changes. If possible, the entire family could be targeted in the recommendations to improve family health to avoid stigmatisation of the overweight child. Golan, Fainaru and Weizman (1998) have shown that, in 5- to 11-year-old children, directing the education and management advice at the parents is more effective than directing the education at the children. For young children, parents control access to food, how food is prepared, how much time is spent watching television and the opportunity and support for physical activity. This may not be true in older children whose lifestyles offer plenty of access to food outside the home and who must therefore learn to self-control their nutritional habits. The older the child, the smaller the family's influence on success of treatment, but the family environment remains a major influence on diet and activity. The more the whole family becomes involved in the programme and changes their behaviour, the greater the positive changes in the children's environment and the greater the social support will be.

Behavioural modifications

Many studies have shown that behavioural procedures may be helpful in promoting lasting changes in physical activity and eating behaviour (Epstein *et al.*, 1980; Robinson, 1999). Behaviour modification techniques provide concrete skills for the children and their parents to change their eating and activity behaviour and achieve a healthy lifestyle. Several behavioural modification techniques can be applied, such as self-monitoring, stimulus control, goal-setting, positive reinforcement, self-talk, social support, problem-solving, relapse prevention and heath education.

Self-monitoring

Self-monitoring includes self-observation and self-recording. The purpose of self-monitoring is to increase awareness of the actual eating and physical activity behaviours and the factors contributing to them. It includes recording food intake and physical activity in a diary. Children should be instructed to record immediately after the behaviour whenever possible. The food diary should include not only the type and quantity of food eaten, but also the time of the day, where the meal was consumed and which foods they have refused to eat when it was offered. The food diary can be used to target times and places when increased food intake is likely or to identify problem foods that can be reduced or eliminated from the diet. The physical activity diary should include type of activities, duration and intensity. Not only physical activities, but also sedentary activities (e.g. television viewing, playing computer games) should be recorded in the diary. Self-monitoring allows the patient and the therapist to identify unhealthy behaviours that can be potentially changed. Appropriate feedback on the food and activity diary should be provided by the therapist. Weight should also be recorded on a regular basis. To de-emphasise weight change in favour of an emphasis on behaviour change, weekly or even monthly weighings are preferable to recording the weight daily. Weighings should be done at the same time of the day (preferably early morning before breakfast) and in the same light clothing. Weighing may also be misleading in children. As they grow, they may gain weight, but at the same time there may be a decrease in body fat. Monitoring body fat would be a better evaluation tool of treatment success. Body fat can be assessed in clinical practices, but not many children have the opportunity to measure body fat at home. Self-monitoring is considered to be the most important factor in behavioural programmes. Effective and continuous self-monitoring is found to be a good predictor of long-term success (Guare et al., 1989).

Stimulus control

Stimulus control involves identifying and modifying the environmental cues or barriers that are associated with the obese child's unhealthy eating or sedentary behaviour. This involves altering access and establishing new routines. Parents could help their children by limiting all eating to one location (for example sitting down at the dining table with the television turned off), reducing the frequency of meals eaten outside the home, limiting the amount of unhealthy food in the house, putting stop signs at the refrigerator and places where food is stored, buying only those items on their prepared food list (no impulse buying), using smaller plates in order to make normal portions look larger, making second servings more difficult to obtain by serving food in the kitchen rather than at the dining table, not forcing the child to finish the entire meal, delaying dessert for 10 to 15 minutes in order to allow the experience of delayed satiety signals, making low-calorie snack foods readily available and keeping high-calorie foods out of sight and reach. Stimulus control strategies that can be applied by the child are taking smaller bites, chewing food longer, putting the fork down between bites and leaving some food on the plate.

Stimulus control strategies that may help increase physical activity are putting up notes to remember to be physically active, laying out exercise clothes and shoes in the morning as a reminder to walk or jog after school, and making sure bikes are easily accessible and not hidden somewhere in the back of the garage. Strategies that may help decrease sedentary activity are moving the television to a less desirable and less prominent location in the home and limiting access to computer games. Family socialising should be centred around physical activity, trips and walks rather than on food or sedentary behaviours.

Goal-setting

The child should be encouraged to set a weekly nutritional and activity goal and to help to determine the reward for reaching the goal. This is often accompanied by a contract that outlines the terms of rewarding changes in behaviour. Realistic goal-setting and separating short-term goals from long-term goals are important to prevent discouragement. Short-term goals are always easier to achieve than long-term ones and give a good feeling of success and mastery to the obese child. Goals should also be very specific. For example, rather than the goal being 'eating less fatty food' or 'doing more physical activities', which is too general, very specific goals should be set such as 'drinking low-fat milk instead of whole milk' or 'walking the dog each day for 20 minutes'. Choose one nutritional and one activity goal at a time. All necessary changes cannot be made at the same time. Once the first goals have been reached, further changes can be agreed upon. Goals for losing weight often differ between the patient and the therapist. The goals children establish for themselves are often, if not always, far in excess of the results to be expected from even the most effective programmes. The therapist should help the patients to set more realistic short-term weight loss goals.

Positive reinforcement

It is important to motivate the children positively and to reward them for their efforts rather than for the obtained modifications. Positive reinforcement includes verbal praise and attention from the treatment team and family members, but could also be a reward. Rewards should be determined together with the child. The child could make a list of activities, privileges and items that are rewarding to the child and acceptable to the parent. Preferably rewards should encourage further participation in physical activity, such as sporting equipment or a trip to the skating rink. Food, money or expensive items should not be chosen as rewards. Rewards should be achievable within a short and definite period to be able to motivate the child. The goals, the timeline for the attainment of the goal and the agreed reward may be specified in a contract between the child and the parents or the therapist. Parents should learn to be observant, so that they are aware of their children's behaviours and can reward them when appropriate. Material rewards should only be used in the initial phase. Ultimately the healthy behaviour should become self-rewarding or the child should learn to reward him- or herself for doing well.

Self talk

Self talk involves teaching the child to turn negative self-statements into positive ones and helping him/her with the negative remarks that other children make about his/her weight. Having children write down and read positive statements about themselves may help to increase self-esteem. Children should also learn that not reaching their goal once or regaining weight once does not make them a failure. Instead they should learn to tell themselves that they are going to keep on trying and do better the next time.

Social support

Support from family members, friends, treatment group members and treatment staff is a very important determinant of treatment success. Parents should be consistent and avoid mixed messages. Parents should be instructed not to do things in front of their children that they do not want the child to imitate and to model healthy eating and active behaviour that they want their child to repeat. Whenever possible, the entire family should adhere to a similar diet. Parents should organise physical activities and trips with the entire family. Children should be encouraged to be active with a sport partner.

Problem-solving and relapse prevention

Problem-solving involves identifying problem situations that place the child at risk of unhealthy behaviours, and developing strategies and solutions to avoid or successfully cope with these high-risk situations. Discussing high-risk situations (such as holidays, parties and social gatherings) in advance and learning how to cope in these situations may prevent relapse. Occasions for eating, such as meals taken outside the home at restaurants and fast-food outlets and school lunches, should also be discussed in advance with the child. Children should learn to participate in physical activities in potentially difficult situations (such as injury, bad weather, tiredness, lack of training partner) and should be verbally encouraged to participate. In the case of bad weather, children may prefer to be inside watching television rather than playing active games outside. In this case, the therapist should draw the child's attention to the fact that there are plenty of active games or exercises that can be easily done inside. In case of injuries, children find it obvious that it is impossible for them to continue being physically active. This is a typical occasion for relapse. In this case, creative solutions should be found. When the child has a broken arm, it is still possible to do a range of activities such as walking, aerobics and playing hopscotch. Although it is more difficult to find alternatives in the case of a broken leg, resistance exercises while sitting or other sitting activities are still possible. Children should also get help to continue their usual activities after recovery from injury.

Nutritional education

Educating the child and parent in basic nutritional concepts is an important part of dietary treatment. Nutritional information should include education about negative effects of unhealthy eating and the benefits of healthy eating, the components of balanced and healthy nutrition, and healthy and safe nutritional changes. It is also important to teach the children and parents how to interpret food labels so they can compare similar products and make healthy choices. It is useful to emphasise the overall health benefits of eating well rather than focusing solely on weight loss effects. Simply providing nutritional education or prescribing a diet is inadequate. Children and parents should also learn how to implement and practice recommended food changes. They should learn how to, for instance, choose the right products in the supermarket, resist the seduction of commercials, prepare healthy meals and estimate appropriate portion sizes. Children could practice at home what they have learned during the sessions, for example taking a healthy lunch box to school, going to the supermarket and cooking a healthy meal. Success or failure should be discussed at the next session.

Physical activity education

Physical activity education sessions can include education about the benefits of physical activity, the negative effects of television viewing, the importance of physical fitness, the difference between sports and physical activities, the energy expenditure of various exercises, the importance of aerobic and resistance training and which exercises are best for weight control, the importance of stretching, warming-up and cooling-down, the importance of drinking water after or while being physically active, and appropriate hygiene after an exercise session. Parental activity behaviour and their knowledge and attitude towards physical activity should also be improved.

Types of programme

Outpatient versus inpatient treatment

Outpatient treatment is preferable to inpatient treatment for most overweight and obese children. Outpatient treatment is much less expensive and children are not removed from their home environment, which are two disadvantages of inpatient treatment. In the case of severe obesity where outpatient management has proved ineffective, inpatient treatment may sometimes be indicated (Frelut, 2002). The dramatic weight loss due to intensive treatment, the integration into a peer group suffering similar problems, the separation from family conflicts and problems and the permanent support from a professional team which has no negative perceptions of the obese child are important benefits of inpatient treatment. Inpatient treatment does not differ in its general principles from outpatient treatment, except that family involvement may be more difficult depending on the distance between the children's homes and the centre. An alternative to inpatient treatment in a clinical setting is the residential summer camp. A great disadvantage of inpatient treatment is that once children return to their (often obesogenic) home environment, it is very difficult to sustain healthy behaviours (Deforche *et al.*, 2004). During inpatient treatment their behaviours were continuously supervised and controlled by the treatment team. This lack of autonomy makes it difficult to learn to control their behaviours, which is a very important technique for long-term weight maintenance.

Group versus individual treatment

Although there are few data available to compare group versus individual treatment in children, there are more arguments in favour of group treatment. Group therapy has the advantage of lower costs, reaching a larger number of children simultaneously, the support and help from other group members and the interaction with other members. The possibility of meeting children with the same weight problem may be a stimulus to attend treatment sessions. Being part of a group of people with the same problem is sometimes a great motivator to deal with their own problem. Group members act as role models. Techniques to change behaviours and control weight may be more easily accepted when suggested by other group members than when promoted by the therapist. Most interventions in children described in the literature are group treatments including individualised behavioural counselling.

Frequency of sessions and duration of treatment

Results from adult studies suggest that the longer and more intensive treatment programmes are the greater the weight loss and long-term weight loss maintenance (Brownell and Jeffery, 1987). It is likely that longer and more intensive treatments will also be beneficial for treating obese children. Most described interventions start with weekly sessions during the initial treatment phase and cut back during the follow-up period. A review of intervention studies in children and adolescents found that treatment periods lasted between 2 and 14 months and the period of follow-up ranged from 8 months to 10 years (Epstein *et al.*, 1998).

Maintenance of weight loss

Weight control is often a chronic lifelong challenge for obese children and adolescents. Weight regain after successful weight loss is very common. Most children regain weight probably because they relapse to old behaviours. Improving the maintenance of weight loss and preventing relapse is an important challenge facing obesity treatment. Long-term follow-up may be difficult for parent and child. The child may lose interest and it may be financially and logistically difficult for the parents. Often funds for follow-up treatment are not available. Although continued support after initial treatment may be essential for long-term success, few data currently exist regarding the best way to follow up children after weight reduction, or regarding factors associated with long-term maintenance of weight loss in children. Results from a pilot study showed that post-treatment telephone contact appears to have the potential to be an effective maintenance strategy in obese youngsters (Deforche *et al.*, 2005a). Another study showed that both physical activity and nutritional habits play an important role in weight maintenance after initial weight loss in children and that one healthy behaviour cannot compensate for another unhealthy behaviour (Deforche *et al.*, 2005b). A balanced low-fat normal calorie diet in combination with regular physical activity of sufficient intensity may be the most appropriate strategy to maintain weight loss after treatment in children.

References

Amador, M., Ramos, L.T., Morono, M. and Hermelo, M.P. (1990) 'Growth rate reduction during energy restriction in obese adolescents', *Experimental and Clinical Endocrinology*, 96: 73–82.

Ballor, D.L. and Keesey, R.E. (1991) 'A meta-analysis of the factors affecting exercise-induced changes in body mass, fat mass and fat-free mass in males and females', *International Journal of Obesity Related Metabolic Disorders*, 15: 717–26.

Barker, R. and Cooke, B. (1992) 'Diet, obesity and being overweight: a qualitative research study', *Health Education Journal*, 51: 117–21.

Biddle, S., Cavill, N. and Sallis, J. (1998) 'Policy framework for young people and health-enhancing physical activity', in S. Biddle, J. Sallis, N. Cavill (eds) *Young and Active? Young People and Health-Enhancing Physical Activity: Evidence and Implications*, London: Health Education Authority, pp. 3–16.

Birch, L.L. and Davison, K.K. (2001) 'Family environmental factors influencing the developing behavioral controls of food intake and childhood overweight', *Pediatric Clinics of North America*, 48: 893–907.

Birch, L.L. and Fisher, J.O. (1998) 'Development of eating behaviors among children and adolescents', *Pediatrics*, 101: 539–49.

Blair, S.N. and Brodney, S. (1999) 'Effects of physical inactivity and obesity on morbidity and mortality: current evidence and research issues', *Medicine and Science in Sport and Exercise*, 31: S646–62.

Brownell, K.D. and Jeffery, R.W. (1987) 'Improving long-term weight-loss – pushing the limits of treatment', *Behavior Therapy*, 18: 353–74.

Caroli, M. and Burniat, W. (2002) 'Dietary management', in W. Burniat, T. Cole, I. Lissau, E. Poskitt (eds) *Child and Adolescent Obesity. Causes and Consequences, Prevention and Management*, Cambridge: Cambridge University Press, pp. 282–306.

Craig, S., Goldberg, J. and Dietz, W.H. (1996) 'Psychosocial correlates of physical activity among fifth and eight graders', *Preventative Medicine*, 25: 506–13.

Deforche, B., De Bourdeaudhuij, I., Tanghe, A., Hills, A.P. and De Bode, P. (2004) 'Changes in physical activity and psychosocial determinants of physical activity in children and adolescents treated for obesity', *Patient Education and Counselling*, 55: 407–15.

Deforche, B., De Bourdeaudhuij, I., Tanghe, A., Debode, P., Hills, A.P. and Bouckaert, J. (2005a) 'Post-treatment phone contact: a weight maintenance strategy in obese youngsters', *International Journal of Obesity*, 29: 543–6.

Deforche, B., De Bourdeaudhuij, I., Tanghe, A., Debode, P., Hills, A.P. and Bouckaert, J. (2005b) 'Role of physical activity and eating behaviour in long-term weight control after treatment in severely obese children and adolescents', *Acta Paediatrica*, 94: 464–70.

Dietz, W. (1999) 'How to tackle the problem early? The role of education in the prevention of obesity', *International Journal of Obesity Related Metabolic Disorders*, 23(Suppl 4): S7–S9.

Dietz, W.H. (2001) 'Breastfeeding may help prevent childhood obesity', *Journal of the American Medical Association*, 285: 2506–7.

Dietz, W.H., Bandini, L.G. and Gortmaker, S. (1990) 'Epidemiologic and metabolic risk factors for childhood obesity. Prepared for the Fourth Congress on Obesity Research, Vienna, Austria, December 1988', *Klinische Pädiatrie*, 202: 69–72.

Epstein, L.H. (1996) 'Family-based behavioural intervention for obese children', *International Journal of Obesity Related Metabolic Disorders*, 20(Suppl 1): S14–21.

Epstein, L.H. and Squires, S. (1988) *The Stoplight Diet for Children: An Eight-Week Program for Parents and Children*, Boston, MA: Little, Brown and Company.

Epstein, L.H., Wing, R.R., Steranchak, L., Dickson, B. and Michelson, J. (1980) 'Comparison of family-based behavior modification and nutrition education for childhood obesity', *Journal of Pediatric Psychology*, 5: 25–36.

Epstein, L.H., Wing, R.R., Koeske, R., Ossip, D.J. and Beck, S. (1982) 'A comparison of lifestyle change and programmed aerobic exercise on weight and fitness changes in obese children', *Behavior Therapy*, 13: 651–65.

Epstein, L.H., Kuller, L.H., Wing, R.R., Valoski, A.M. and McCurley, J. (1989) 'The effect of weight control on lipid changes in obese children', *American Journal of Diseases of Children*, 143: 454–7.

Epstein, L.H., Smith, J.A., Vara, L.S. and Rodefer, J.S. (1991) 'Behavioral economic analysis of activity choice in obese children', *Health Psychology*, 10: 311–16.

Epstein, L.H., Valoski, A.M., Vara, L.S., McCurley, J., Wisniewski, L., Kalarchian, M.A., Klein, K.R. and Shrager, L.R. (1995a) 'Effects of decreasing sedentary behavior and increasing activity on weight change in obese children', *Health Psychology*, 14: 109–15.

Epstein, L.H., Valoski, A.M., Kalarchian, M.A. and McCurley, J. (1995b) 'Do children lose and maintain weight easier than adults – a comparison of child and parent weight changes from 6 months to 10 years', *Obesity Research*, 5: 411–17.

Epstein, L.H., Myers, M.D., Raynor, H.A. and Saelens, B.E. (1998) 'Treatment of pediatric obesity', *Pediatrics*, 101: 554–70.

Evers, C. (1997) 'Empower children to develop healthful eating habits', *Journal of the American Dietetics Association*, 97(Suppl 2): S116–18.

Fogelholm, M., Nuutinen, O., Pasanen, M., Myohanen, E. and Saatela, T. (1999) 'Parent–child relationship of physical activity patterns and obesity', *International Journal of Obesity Related Metabolic Disorders*, 23: 1262–5.

Frelut, M.-L. (2002) 'Interdisciplinary residential management', in W. Burniat, T. Cole, I. Lissau, E. Poskitt (eds) *Child and Adolescent Obesity. Causes and Consequences, Prevention and Management*, Cambridge: Cambridge University Press, pp. 377–88.

Fulton, J.E., McGuire, M.T., Caspersen, C.J. and Dietz, W.H. (2001) 'Interventions for weight loss and weight gain prevention among youth: current issues', *Sports Medicine*, 31: 153–65.

Golan, M., Fainaru, M. and Weizman, A. (1998) 'Role of behaviour modification in the treatment of childhood obesity with the parents as the exclusive agents of change', *International Journal of Obesity Related Metabolic Disorders*, 22: 1217–24.

Grace, C.M. (2001) 'Dietary management of obesity', in P.G. Kopelman (ed.) *Management of Obesity and Related Disorders*, London: Martin Dunitz Ltd, pp. 129–64.

Grilo, C.M. (1994) 'Physical activity and obesity', *Biomedicine and Pharmacotherapy*, 48: 127–36.

Guare, J.C., Wing, R.R., Marcus, M.D., Epstein, L.H., Burton, L.R. and Gooding, W.E. (1989) 'Analysis of changes in eating behavior and weight loss in type II diabetic patients. Which behaviors to change', *Diabetes Care*, 12: 500–3.

Hodges, E.A. (2003) 'A primer on early childhood obesity and parental influence', *Pediatric Nursing*, 29: 13–16.

Jakicic, J.M. (2002) 'The role of physical activity in prevention and treatment of body weight gain in adults', *Journal of Nutrition*, 132: S3826–9.

Kelder, S.H., Perry, C.L., Klepp, K.I. and Lytle, L.L. (1994) 'Longitudinal tracking of adolescent smoking, physical activity, and food choice behaviours', *American Journal of Public Health*, 84: 1121–6.

Kraak, V. and Pelletier, D.L. (1998) 'The influence of commercialism on the food purchase behavior of children and teenage youth', *Family Economics and Nutrition Reviews*, 11: 15–23.

McLean, N., Griffin, S., Toney, K. and Hardeman, W. (2003) 'Family involvement in weight control, weight maintenance and weight-loss interventions: a systematic review of randomised trials', *International Journal of Obesity Related Metabolic Disorders*, 27: 987–1005.

Maffeis, C., Schutz, Y. and Pinelli, L. (1992) 'Effect of weight loss on resting energy expenditure in obese prepubertal children', *International Journal of Obesity Related Metabolic Disorders*, 16: 41–7.

Pidlich, J., Pfeffel, F., Zwiauer, K., Schneider, B. and Schmindinger, H. (1997) 'The effect of weight reduction on the surface electrocardiogram: a prospective trial in obese children and adolescents', *International Journal of Obesity Related Metabolic Disorders*, 21: 1018–23.

Power, C., Lake, J.K. and Cole, T.J. (1997) 'Measurement and longterm health risks of child and adolescent fatness', *International Journal of Obesity Related Metabolic Disorders*, 21: 507–26.

Robinson, T.N. (1999) 'Behavioural treatment of childhood and adolescent obesity', *International Journal of Obesity Related Metabolic Disorders*, 23 (Suppl 2): S52–7.

Rolland-Cachera, M.F. and Bellisle, F. (2002) 'Nutrition', in W. Burniat, T. Cole, I. Lissau, E. Poskitt (eds.) *Child and Adolescent Obesity. Causes and Consequences, Prevention and Management*, Cambridge: Cambridge University Press, pp. 69–92.

Saris, W.H., Blair, S.N., van Baak, M.A., Eaton, S.B., Davies, P.S., Di Pietro, L., Fogelholm, M., Rissanen, A., Schoeller, D., Swinburn, B., Tremblay, A., Westerterp, K.R. and Wyatt, H. (2003) 'How much physical activity is enough to prevent unhealthy weight gain? Outcome of the IASO 1st Stock Conference and consensus statement', *Obesity Reviews*, 4: 101–14.

Schonfeld-Warden, N. and Warden, C.H. (1997) 'Pediatric obesity: an overview of etiology and treatment', *Pediatric Clinics of North America*, 44: 339–61.

Sothern, M.S., Loftin, J.M., Udall, J.N., Suskind, R.M., Ewing, T.L., Tang, S.C. and Blecker, U. (1999) 'Inclusion of resistence exercise in a multidisciplinary outpatient treatment program for preadolescent obese children', *Southern Medical Journal*, 92: 585–92.

Stallings, V., Archibald, E., Pencharz, P., Harrison, J. and Bell, L. (1988) 'One-year follow-up of weight, total body potassium, and total body nitrogen in obese adolescents treated with the protein-sparing modified fast', *American Journal of Clinical Nutrition*, 48: 91–4.

Story, M. (1999) 'School-based approaches for preventing and treating obesity', *International Journal of Obesity Related Metabolic Disorders*, 23(Suppl 2): S43–51.

Tremblay, A., Doucet, E. and Imbeault, P. (1999) 'Physical activity and weight maintenance', *International Journal of Obesity Related Metabolic Disorders*, 23(Suppl 3): S50–4.

Treuth, M.S., Hunter, G.R., Pichon, C., Figueroa-Colon, R. and Goran, M.I. (1998) 'Fitness and energy expenditure after strength training in obese prepubertal girls', *Medicine and Science in Sports and Exercise*, 30: 1130–6.

Widhalm, L. and Zwiauer, K. (1987) 'Metabolic effects of a very low calorie diet in obese children and adolescents with special reference to nitrogen balance', *Journal of the American College of Nutrition*, 6: 467–74.

Zwiauer, K.F.M. (2000) 'Prevention and treatment of overweight and obesity in children and adolescents', *European Journal of Pediatrics*, 159(Suppl 1): S56–68.

Index